Edward R. Canda, PhD
Elizabeth D. Smith, DSW
Editors

Transpersonal Perspectives on Spirituality in Social Work

Transpersonal Perspectives on Spirituality in Social Work has been co-published simultaneously as *Social Thought*, Volume 20, Numbers 1/2 2001.

Pre-publication
REVIEWS,
COMMENTARIES,
EVALUATIONS . . .

"**C**OMPREHENSIVE . . . provides theoretical and practice-oriented studies on the emerging field of transpersonal social work. The writing is both scholarly and relevant to practice. OF INTEREST TO SCHOLARS, PRACTITIONERS, AND STUDENTS ALIKE."

John R. Graham, PhD, RSW
Associate Professor
Faculty of Social Work
University of Calgary
Alberta, Canada

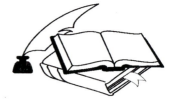

Transpersonal Perspectives on Spirituality in Social Work

Transpersonal Perspectives on Spirituality in Social Work has been co-published simultaneously as *Social Thought*, Volume 20, Numbers 1/2 2001.

The *Social Thought* Monographic ''Separates''

Below is a list of " separates," which in serials librarianship means a special issue simultaneously published as a special journal issue or double-issue *and* as a "separate" hardbound monograph. (This is a format which we also call a "DocuSerial.")

"Separates" are published because specialized libraries or professionals may wish to purchase a specific thematic issue by itself in a format which can be separately cataloged and shelved, as opposed to purchasing the journal on an on-going basis. Faculty members may also more easily consider a "separate" for classroom adoption.

"Separates" are carefully classified separately with the major book jobbers so that the journal tie-in can be noted on new book order slips to avoid duplicate purchasing.

You may wish to visit Haworth's Website at . . .

http://www.HaworthPress.com

. . . to search our online catalog for complete tables of contents of these separates and related publications.

You may also call 1-800-HAWORTH (outside US/Canada: 607-722-5857), or Fax 1-800-895-0582 (outside US/Canada: 607-771-0012), or e-mail at:

getinfo@haworthpressinc.com

Transpersonal Perspectives on Spirituality in Social Work, edited by Edward R. Canda, PhD, and Elizabeth D. Smith, DSW (Vol. 20, No. 1/2, 2001). *"COMPREHENSIVE. . . provides theoretical and practice-oriented studies on the emerging field of transpersonal social work. The writing is both scholarly and relevant to practice. OF INTEREST TO SCHOLARS, PRACTITIONERS, AND STUDENTS ALIKE." (John R. Graham, PhD, RSW, Associate Professor, Faculty of Social Work, University of Calgary, Alberta, Canada)*

Raising Our Children Out of Poverty, edited by John J. Stretch, PhD, Maria Bartlett, PhD, William J. Hutchison, PhD, Susan A. Taylor, PhD, and Jan Wilson, MSW (Vol. 19, No. 2, 1999). *This book shows what can be done at the national and local community levels to raise children out of poverty by strengthening families, communities, and social services.*

Postmodernism, Religion and the Future of Social Work, edited by Roland G. Meinert, PhD, John T. Pardeck, PhD, and John W. Murphy, PhD (Vol. 18, No. 3, 1998). *"Critically important for social work as it attempts to effectively respond to its increasingly complex roles and demands. . . . A book worth owning and studying." (John M. Herrick, PhD, Acting Director, School of Social Work, Michigan State University, East Lansing, Michigan)*

Spirituality in Social Work: New Directions, edited by Edward R. Canda, PhD (Vol. 18, No. 2, 1998). *"Provides interesting insights and references for those who seek to develop curricula responsive to the spiritual challenges confronting our profession and the populations we serve." (Au-Deane S. Cowley, PhD, Associate Dean, Graduate School of Social Work, University of Utah, Salt Lake City)*

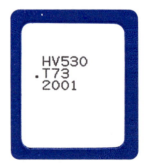

Transpersonal Perspectives on Spirituality in Social Work

Edward R. Canda
Elizabeth D. Smith
Editors

Transpersonal Perspectives on Spirituality in Social Work has been co-published simultaneously as *Social Thought*, Volume 20, Numbers 1/2 2001.

The Haworth Press, Inc.
and The Haworth Pastoral Press,
an Imprint of The Haworth Press, Inc.
New York • London • Oxford

Transpersonal Perspectives on Spirituality in Social Work has been co-published simultaneously as *Social Thought*™, Volume 20, Numbers 1/2 2001.

The development, preparation, and publication of this work has been undertaken with great care. However, the publisher, employees, editors, and agents of The Haworth Press and all imprints of The Haworth Press, Inc., including The Haworth Medical Press® and Pharmaceutical Products Press®, are not responsible for any errors contained herein or for consequences that may ensue from use of materials or information contained in this work. Opinions expressed by the author(s) are not necessarily those of The Haworth Press, Inc.

The Haworth Press, Inc., 10 Alice Street, Binghamton, NY 13904-1580 USA

Cover design by Thomas J. Mayshock Jr.

Library of Congress Cataloging-in-Publication Data

Transpersonal Perspectives on Spirituality in Social Work / Edward R. Canda, and Elizabeth D. Smith editors.
     p. cm.
     "Co-published simultaneously as Social thought, volume 20, numbers 1/2 2001."
     Includes bibliographical references and index.
     ISBN 0-7890-1394-0 (alk. paper) – ISBN 0-7890-1395-9 (alk. paper)
     1. Social Service–Religious Aspects. 2. Spirituality. I. Canda, Edward R. II. Smith, Elizabeth D. III. Social thought.
HV530 .T73 2001
361.3′2–dc21
                                                 2001039145

Indexing, Abstracting & Website/Internet Coverage

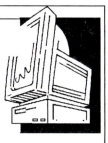

This section provides you with a list of major indexing & abstracting services. That is to say, each service began covering this periodical during the year noted in the right column. Most Websites which are listed below have indicated that they will either post, disseminate, compile, archive, cite or alter their own Website users with research-based content from this work. (This list is as current as the copyright date of this publication.)

(continued)

Special Bibliographic Notes related to special journal issues (separates) and indexing/abstracting:

- indexing/abstracting services in this list will also cover material in any "separate" that is co-published simultaneously with Haworth's special thematic journal issue or DocuSerial. Indexing/abstracting usually covers material at the article/chapter level.
- monographic co-editions are intended for either non-subscribers or libraries which intend to purchase a second copy for their circulating collections.
- monographic co-editions are reported to all jobbers/wholesalers/approval plans. The source journal is listed as the "series" to assist the prevention of duplicate purchasing in the same manner utilized for books-in-series.
- to facilitate user/access services all indexing/abstracting services are encouraged to utilize the co-indexing entry note indicated at the bottom of the first page of each article/chapter/contribution.
- this is intended to assist a library user of any reference tool (whether print, electronic, online, or CD-ROM) to locate the monographic version if the library has purchased this version but not a subscription to the source journal.
- individual articles/chapters in any Haworth publication are also available through the Haworth Document Delivery Service (HDDS).

Transpersonal Perspectives on Spirituality in Social Work

CONTENTS

ABOUT THE EDITORS

Edward R. Canda, PhD, is Professor in and Chairperson of the doctoral program at the University of Kansas School of Social Welfare, Lawrence, KS 66045. He is also a member of the Center for East Asian Studies and a coordinator of the linkage between religious studies and social work educational programs at the University of Kansas. He has more than 50 publications on the topics of spirituality and cultural diversity in social work. More than 100 presentations span North America, Europe, and East Asia. His most recent book is *Spiritual Diversity in Social Work Practice: The Heart of Helping*, co-authored with Leola Dyrud Furman, published by Free Press in 1999. In 1990, Dr. Canda founded the Society for Spirituality and Social Work.

Elizabeth D. Smith, DSW, is Associate Professor in and Chairperson of the doctoral program at the National Catholic School of Social Service, The Catholic University of America, Washington, DC 20064. She also holds a part-time faculty position of Research Associate at Johns Hopkins University, School of Medicine. Over the past fifteen years her research has centered on spirituality and death, in particular suffering and the process of confronting one's mortality. Dr. Smith has presented nationally and internationally on these topics and is currently in the process of writing a book entitled *The Transformation of Suffering: A Transpersonal Body, Mind and Spirit Model of Social Work Practice*. She is Vice-President of the Society for Spirituality and Social Work.

Introduction

Edward R. Canda
Elizabeth D. Smith

KEYWORDS. Spirituality, transpersonal, religion, social work, psychology

The groundbreaking topic of transpersonal social work presented herein is especially apropos for social work early in this new millennium, as transpersonal theory calls us to go beyond the limits and biases of egoistic and ethnocentric views of the self, the world, well-being, and justice.

As will be shown in the following chapters, transpersonal theory has been growing steadily within psychology and philosophy since the 1960s and has gained tremendous momentum since the 1990s. However, it has only recently begun to influence mainstream social work. *Transpersonal Perspectives on Spirituality in Social Work* is intended to stimulate a quantum leap in social work innovation by helping scholars and practitioners to incorporate the important contributions of transpersonal thought and practice. For this purpose, we have collected a set of theoretical and practice oriented studies that establish a foundation for the newly emerging field of transpersonal social work. Transpersonal theory brings us back to ideas about spiritual aspects of human needs that inspired the foundation of American social work. At the same time, it

---

Edward R. Canda, PhD, is Professor in and Chairperson of the doctoral program at the University of Kansas School of Social Welfare, Lawrence, KS 66045.

Elizabeth D. Smith, DSW, is Associate Professor and Chairperson of the doctoral program at the National Catholic School of Social Service, The Catholic University of America, Washington, DC 20064.

[Haworth co-indexing entry note]: "Introduction." Canda, Edward R., and Elizabeth D. Smith. Co-published simultaneously in *Social Thought* (The Haworth Press, Inc.) Vol. 20, No. 1/2, 2001, pp. 1-3; and: *Transpersonal Perspectives on Spirituality in Social Work* (ed: Edward R. Canda, and Elizabeth D. Smith) The Haworth Press, Inc., 2001, pp. 1-3. Single or multiple copies of this article are available for a fee from The Haworth Document Delivery Service [1-800-342-9678, 9:00 a.m. - 5:00 p.m. (EST). E-mail address: getinfo@haworthpressinc.com].

1

propels us into challenging new perspectives derived from diverse scientific fields, Western and Eastern philosophies, and ancient and emerging worldviews.

We have organized the contents to flow from conceptual and theoretical frameworks for understanding transpersonal theory to empirical and clinical studies that focus on people's actual life experiences and social work practice implications.

Carroll's comparative analysis of various models of spirituality and spiritual development sets the context of concern for transpersonal social work, which is to address the full range of human potential from material and psychological well-being to spiritual fulfillment. Besthorn offers insights about the fundamental connectedness between human being and nature in the person/environment whole by weaving together contributions of transpersonal theory and deep ecology. Smith addresses universal human concerns about mortality and death and suggests how social workers can help alleviate death-related anxiety by applying a transpersonal and social constructionist approach. Leight points out ways that transpersonal theory can complement and enhance social work practice that focuses on empowerment and justice in work with marginalized and oppressed populations.

Cowley shows how social workers, particularly in mental health settings, can develop guidelines for differentiating between psychopathology-based hallucinations or delusions and spiritual breakthroughs of consciousness. Freeman's study explores differences in archetypes of spiritual significance between European Americans and African Americans and how they relate to expressions of violence. Canda's study of adults with a chronic illness gives a detailed example of how people can draw on transpersonal experiences and beliefs to support resilient response to challenges related to disability and death. Reese gives theoretical, empirical, and practical insights into transpersonally oriented hospice work. Finally, Derezotes provides a model for promoting compatibility and intimacy through transpersonally oriented clinical practice with couples.

All together, these articles take us through the full sweep of human experience from depths of crisis, illness, death, and injustice to peaks of spiritual illumination and transformation. Looking at this sweep of human experience more closely through the lens of transpersonal theory, social workers can perceive how spiritual growth and development are actually happening through all the lows and highs of life. Then we can align our work with this sacred process in accord with the particular spiritual traditions and practices of our clients and ourselves.

We believe that this book is groundbreaking in the profession of social work in that it presents both explanatory insights of transpersonal theory and also their implications for promoting growth and change through practice that is relevant to social work's unique person-in-environment perspective. The development of models of practice that employ transpersonal theory and the application of holistic theoretical concepts to social work is long overdue. It is our hope that this work will spawn further research and numerous applications of the transpersonal perspective such that the fourth dimension of the individual, the spiritual, becomes a natural extension of the bio-psycho-social approach.

Furthermore, we hope that this book triggers a conversation in the social work literature about the strengths and limitations of transpersonal theory for exploring spiritual growth-related phenomena and transegoic experiences. In the past, the creative usefulness of these experiences has been neglected due to the limits of conventional Western psychology's materialistic focus on modifying the personality, primarily through talk therapy. Transpersonal theory offers the profession a whole new realm for possible helping strategies and practices and a myriad of methodologies for accessing the spiritual dimension without the imposition of a particular set of beliefs. We invite you to explore the numerous possibilities apparent in each of the articles that might encourage you to extend your own practice, teaching, and/or research.

An edition such as this does not come into being without the cooperative efforts of a number of individuals. Dr. Elizabeth D. Smith gave birth to this project out of her desire to introduce transpersonal theory into the social work literature as a viable option for holistic social work practice. As the primary editor, Dr. Edward R. Canda took the collective body of this work and worked closely with the contributing authors to shape it into a cohesive whole. And behind the scenes, Dr. Fred Ahearn, Editor of *Social Thought*, provided generous help as a skillful reviewer and text editor, for which we extend our gratitude and thanks. We thank the many manuscript reviewers, as well as Marian Abegg, who gave extensive assistance with manuscript preparation. Finally, we thank the contributing authors who are at the forefront of innovation about transpersonal theory and practice in social work.

Conceptual Models of Spirituality

Maria M. Carroll

SUMMARY. The traditional social work view of human nature and the whole person has emphasized biological, psychological, and social dimensions. Interdisciplinary and, more recently, social work conceptualizations of the whole person have added spirituality. After exploring definitions of spirituality, this article describes seven models which include diagrams that enhance the conceptual understanding of spirituality. The models are examined with regard to the spiritual growth process by drawing on developmental theories. A new diagrammatic model, Spirituality: A Wholistic Model, illustrates the relationship between spirituality and the biological, psychological, social, and transpersonal dimensions of the person. It provides a way to evaluate the helpfulness of experiences, including practice interventions, with respect to their role in assisting each individual in moving toward realization of full potential. *[Article copies available for a fee from The Haworth Document Delivery Service: 1-800-342-9678. E-mail address: <getinfo@haworthpressinc.com> Website: <http://www.HaworthPress.com> © 2001 by The Haworth Press, Inc. All rights reserved.]*

KEYWORDS. Spirituality, development, transpersonal, conceptual models, social work

Maria M. Carroll, PhD, LCSW, is Associate Professor in the Department of Social Work at Delaware State University, Dover, DE 19904-2277 (E-mail: MCarrol@dsc.edu).

[Haworth co-indexing entry note]: "Conceptual Models of Spirituality." Carroll, Maria M. Co-published simultaneously in *Social Thought* (The Haworth Press, Inc.) Vol. 20, No. 1/2, 2001, pp. 5-21; and: *Transpersonal Perspectives on Spirituality in Social Work* (ed: Edward R. Canda, and Elizabeth D. Smith) The Haworth Press, Inc., 2001, pp. 5-21. Single or multiple copies of this article are available for a fee from The Haworth Document Delivery Service [1-800-342-9678, 9:00 a.m. - 5:00 p.m. (EST). E-mail address: getinfo@haworthpressinc.com].

CONCEPTUAL MODELS OF SPIRITUALITY

Some helping professions such as social work (Corbett, 1925; Keith-Lucas, 1960; O'Brien, 1992; Richmond, 1930; Siporin, 1985) and nursing (Carson, 1989a; Stoll, 1989) historically have emphasized the whole person. However, they have usually emphasized the biological, psychological, and social dimensions of personhood while minimizing spirituality.

As spirituality has been increasingly considered essential for understanding the whole person, social work literature has broadened its focus to include it (e.g., Bullis, 1996; Canda, 1986, 1988a, 1997; Carroll, 1997b; Cornett, 1992; Cowley, 1993; Weick, 1983b). This new focus has raised questions such as: What is spirituality? What is the relationship between spirituality, clients' experiences, and the idea of the whole person or wholeness? How are the elements of wholeness related? How is spiritual growth demonstrated?

Spirituality, in its broadest sense, has been described as relationship or interconnectedness among self, others, and God–among all that exists in the universe (Canda, 1983). Models depicting wholeness, therefore, include the various dimensions of the person and show their interrelatedness according to the particular theorist's view. In addition to discussing spirituality and wholeness in conceptual models, several theorists from various disciplines have diagramed their models. These visual representations enhance the understanding of conceptual models.

This article will define spirituality in two different ways, present seven diagrammatic models which include spirituality, and discuss spiritual development as a process of growth toward wholeness. It will then present a new diagrammatic model of spirituality which includes its two most common meanings as well as a wholistic developmental perspective.

MEANINGS OF SPIRITUALITY

Descriptions of spirituality contain various themes. One theme is a person's experiential knowledge of and relationship with a transcendent and ultimate source of reality or creation (Berenson, 1987; Bullis, 1996; Fowler, 1981; Siporin, 1985; Titone, 1991). This relationship with God, or the transcendent, is described as a person's openness and responsiveness to God (Helminiak, 1987), sense of well-being in relation to God (the religious component) (Ellison, 1983), and focus on ultimate reality (Canda & Furman, 1999). This relationship with the transcendent may (but not necessarily) be expressed through organized religion, which serves as a means to express one's beliefs about his or her spiritual nature (Dudley & Helfgott, 1990; Ortiz, 1991; Titone, 1991).

A second theme refers to spirituality originating from the deepest core of the person (Canda, 1990; Jung, 1954a; Siporin, 1985). This is described as what is given as a birthright (Helminiack, 1987), one's fundamental nature (Ortiz, 1991), "the ground of our being" (Joseph, 1988, p. 444), soul (Siporin, 1985), and an intangible, life-giving principle or force (Stoll, 1989).

These themes are interrelated and complementary (Canda, 1990, 1997). In discussing social work's conceptualization of spirituality, Carroll (1998) identified two different meanings of spirituality: spirituality-as-essence and spirituality-as-one-dimension. "Spirituality-as-essence refers to a core nature which provides the motivating energy toward meeting the potential for self-development and self-transformation [whereas] . . . spirituality-as-one-dimension refers specifically to one's search for meaning and relationship with God, the transcendent, or ultimate reality" (p. 11). Spirituality-as-one-dimension is frequently considered to be the "transpersonal" dimension of a person. The dimension of relatedness to God and the transcendent (however that relationship is expressed) may be framed within or separate from the belief system of an organized religion. Various words–God, transcendent, and others (e.g., creator, Higher Power, life energy)–will be used interchangeably in referring to relationship with the transpersonal. These two themes, the transpersonal dimension and spirituality (-as-essence), set the stage for exploring wholeness as reflected in diagrammatic models.

DIAGRAMMATIC MODELS OF SPIRITUALITY

From earlier world views of a heaven-earth relationship, Ellison (1983) developed a model called here the Vertical-Horizontal Approach (see Figure 1). It is indicated by two intersecting lines which represent two different, but interrelated, dimensions. The first dimension is relationship directly with God (or however the transcendent is conceptualized), and the second is all other relationships–with self, others, and the environment. While most writers discuss both of these dimensions, Ellison (1983) goes a step further by specifically identifying their separateness and interrelatedness. Although not actually constructing a diagram, he explicitly describes these dimensions as directional: *vertical and horizontal*. The *vertical* dimension refers to the relationship with God or the transcendent which is beyond and/or outside of self and is the source of the supreme values which guide one's life. The *horizontal* dimension refers to the kind and quality of one's relationships with self and others, to well-being in relation to self and others, and to a sense of life purpose and satis-

FIGURE 1. Vertical-horizontal approach as described by Ellison (1983). Constructed by author.

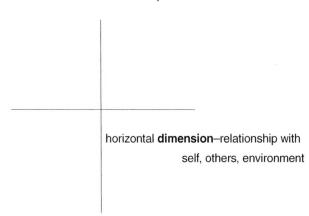

faction. This dimension may be described as the social-psychological component.

Sometimes the two dimensions are inextricably intertwined. For instance, spirituality is described as experiential awareness of transcendent realities which is reflected by the center of value in one's life and by the quality of one's relationships with the universe/God (Ellison, 1983) and as "union with the immanent, supernatural powers that guide people and the universe for good or evil" (Siporin, 1985, p. 210). When spirituality refers to human relationships and life's activities, it refers to manifestations of one's relationship with God; the horizontal dimension, therefore, seems to require and reflect the vertical.

The second model is a series of concentric circles that reflect five levels of consciousness (see Figure 2) (Vaughan, 1985/1995). (Although originally untitled, this model will be identified here as Five Levels of Consciousness.) The innermost circle is the physical dimension; moving outward, the other successive levels are the emotional, mental, existential, and spiritual. Outside of these five circles or levels (and not encircled or limited) is Absolute Spirit or "the underlying ground of the psyche" (Vaughan, 1995, p. 20). Each level involves acceptance and observation. Awareness of the outer levels requires that the preceding levels be relatively calm. "Although health or pathology at each level may appear to be independent of other levels, healing the whole person depends on awareness of well-being on all of them" (p. 21).

FIGURE 2. Five levels of consciousness. Reprinted from Vaughan, Frances (1985/1995). *The Inward Arc: Healing in Psychotherapy and Spirituality* (2nd ed.), Nevada City, CA: Blue Dolphin Publishing, p. 22. Copyright 1985, 1995 Frances E. Vaughan. Used by permission.

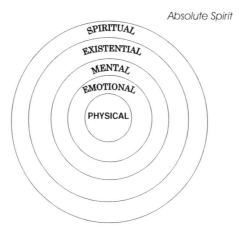

Farran, Fitchett, Quiring-Emblen, and Burck (1989) acknowledge a substantive definition of spirituality which is grounded in the belief in a transcendent and universal being or force. However, they also use a functional definition of spirituality as the person's ultimate commitment or value due to the human need to find meaning. They propose the third and fourth models to be considered here (see Figure 3). The Integrated Approach considers the spiritual dimension as one aspect equal with other dimensions (physiological, psychological, and sociological) of the person whereas the Unifying Approach views the spiritual dimension as a "totality" underlying, embracing, and unifying the other parts of the person.

A fifth model, developed by Kilpatrick and Holland (1990), is called the Self-Other-Context-Spiritual (SOCS) Circle (see Figure 4). The four realities or areas encompass all which exists or is experienced; each of the four areas needs to be fully recognized for optimal functioning. "Self" refers to the subjective reality; "other" refers to the external world of objects and states; "context" refers to "the world in the objective sense" (p. 132); and "spiritual" refers to God or the universal governing force. Three of the dimensions (self, other, and context) form a triangle within a circle. By surrounding the triangle, the spiritual dimension encompasses, permeates, and integrates the other three areas. The spiritual dimension contains two components: (1) values which provide

FIGURE 3. Options for viewing the spiritual dimension. Reprinted from "Development of a Model for Spiritual Assessment and Intervention," by C. F. Ferran, G. Fitchett, J. D. Quiring-Emblen, & J. R. Burck, 1989, *Journal of Religion & Health*, 28(3), p. 29. Copyright 1989 by Institutes of Religion and Health, Inc. Reprinted with permission.

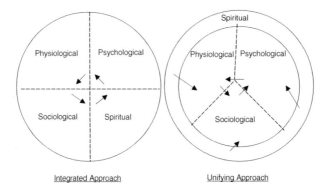

FIGURE 4. SOCS circle presentation of the Four Life Realities. Reprinted from "Spiritual Dimensions of Practice," by A. C. Kilpatrick and T. P. Holland, 1990, *The Clinical Supervisor*, 8, p. 133. Copyright 1990 by The Haworth Press, Inc. Reprinted with permission.

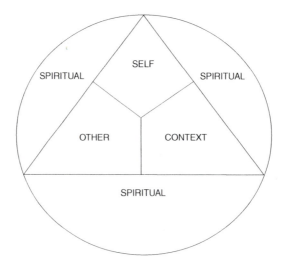

meaning, worth, and direction; and (2) faith which provides a way of understanding life.

The sixth model, A Holistic Model of Spirituality (Canda & Furman, 1999), consists of three concentric circles (see Figure 5). The inner circle is the center of the person, the middle circle is divided into quadrants (biological, psychological, sociological, and spiritual aspects), and the outer circle is the wholeness of the person in relationship with all. In this model, there are three metaphors for spirituality. In the middle circle, spirituality refers to the spiritual aspect of the person, which complements the other three aspects. It involves a search for meaning and morally fulfilling relations with self, others, and ultimate reality, however a person defines it. The outer circle represents

FIGURE 5. A holistic model of spirituality. Reprinted from E. R. Canda and L. D. Furman, 1999, *Spiritual Diversity in Social Work Practice*, New York: The Free Press, p. 46. Copyright 1999 Edward R. Canda, PhD, & Leola Dyrud Furman, PhD. Reprinted with permission.

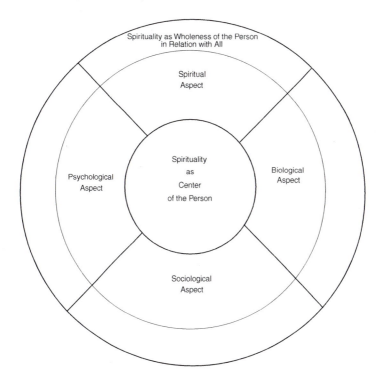

spirituality as wholeness of the person in relation with all. It transcends and embraces the four aspects of a person. The center circle represents spirituality as the center of the person. It is immanent within the person and integrates all aspects.

The seventh model, The Whole Person: A Model (Ellor, Netting, & Thibault, 1999), is three-dimensional (see Figure 6). The spiritual dimension (on the top level) includes affective, behavioral, and cognitive aspects; the traditional clinical dimensions (on the bottom level) include the physical, emotional, and social dimensions. The in-between space, Integrative Dimension, provides the vehicle through which the Spiritual Dimension interacts with the traditional dimensions.

All of these models reflect the whole person and his or her dimensions but do so in different ways depending on the definition or meaning of spirituality. *Spirituality as soul, essence, or ground of one's being* is present in A Holistic Model of Spirituality (as Center of the Person) and in The Whole Person: A Model (in the Integrative Dimension). It is also implied in the Vertical-Horizontal Approach (both axes together), in the SOCS Circle (with values and faith originating from one's core), in the spiritual dimension of the Unifying Approach (with the basic need to find meaning originating from one's core), and in the Absolute Spirit of the Five Levels of Consciousness.

The *transpersonal dimension* is reflected in the vertical axis of Vertical-Horizontal Approach, in the spiritual level of Vaughan's (1995) model

FIGURE 6. The whole person: A model. Reprinted from Ellor, James W., Netting, F. Ellen, & Thibault, Jane M. (1999). *Understanding Religious and Spiritual Aspects of Human Service Practice*, Columbia, SC: University of South Carolina Press, p. 118.

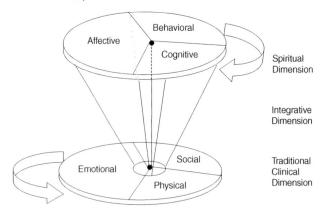

(with five levels of consciousness), in the spiritual aspect of A Holistic Model of Spirituality, and in the spiritual dimension of The Whole Person: A Model. This concept is not explicitly included in the Unifying Approach although implicitly such a relationship may be important if not essential in the human need to find meaning (as Farran et al. (1989) define spirituality). Similarly, with respect to the SOCS Circle, such a relationship is implicitly included if the relationship provides a way of finding meaning through values and faith. Descriptions of spirituality as manifestations of relationship with God or the transcendent are seen in the horizontal axis of the Vertical Approach and in the spiritual dimension of the SOCS Circle through the use of values and faith. Relationship with the transcendent is also seen in the spiritual dimension of the Integrated and Unifying Approaches with respect to values if the ultimate commitment is to the transcendent. This relationship is also evident in the traditional dimensions of The Whole Person: A Model through the action of the integrative dimension and is implied in all three metaphors for spirituality in a Holistic Model of Spirituality.

GROWTH TOWARD WHOLENESS

Common to both themes (of spirituality as one dimension and as a person's essence) is the goal of wholeness which includes all aspects of self-physical, emotional, mental, social, and transpersonal (Canda, 1990, 1997; Fowler, 1981; Jung, 1954a; Maslow, 1967/1971; Sermabeikian, 1994; Vaughan, 1995). However, the process of moving toward wholeness is not always addressed or is done so in very different ways.

Growth in the Transpersonal Dimension

This conscious relationship with the transcendent emerges from an experiential awareness which may occur at any time and in various ways including moments of insight.

The Integrated and Unifying Approaches and the SOCS Circle address the nature of the whole person but do not discuss the process toward wholeness. Through its successive levels, the Five Levels of Consciousness model outlines a growth process in the sense that each of the levels needs to be developed; however, the growth may not occur in a sequential order. Growth in one's inner life (the existential and spiritual levels) may occur along with growth in the other levels; in fact, the two may enhance each other (Vaughan, 1995).

The Vertical-Horizontal Approach is described and diagramed in such a way potentially to reflect growth of either dimension even though one's relationship with self and others (horizontal dimension) seems to require and reflect one's relationship with God or the transcendent (the vertical dimension). Independent development of the psycho-social dimensions, however, may occur when there is a lack of awareness or an unconsciousness of God or the transcendent. This rationale would support Carson (1989a) who says that either dimension can develop completely independently of the other.

In A Holistic Model of Spirituality, the spiritual aspect provides meaning and purpose. It points people toward things that have ultimate value. In The Whole Person: A Model, the (affective, behavioral, and cognitive) aspects of the spiritual dimension provide ways through which the person connects with a larger reality. This connection then influences the traditional clinical dimensions through the integrative dimension.

Descriptions of these models and the growth process focus primarily on one's relationship with God or the transcendent and its reflection in one's relationship with self and others. Another focus, distinct from growth in the transpersonal dimension, is growth or development of one's spiritual or core nature.

Growth of One's Essence or Spirituality

Jung (1933) and Fowler (1981) view spirituality as a person's soul or essence which contains a potential needing to be fulfilled through a developmental process. In addition, spirituality provides the energy for this life-long process, beginning at birth, of actualizing and realizing one's potential (Jung, 1934/1954a). This process potentially culminates in personality completion or wholeness with increasing consciousness of transcendent realities and increasingly greater connectedness with self, others, and all in the universe. Specific conceptual developmental models include Jung's theory of personality development (Jung, 1933; 1934/1954a), Maslow's hierarchy of needs (Maslow, 1962, 1971), Fowler's faith development theory (Fowler, 1981), the structural-hierarchical or transpersonal spectrum model (Wilber, Engler, & Brown, 1986), and the dynamic-dialectical paradigm (Washburn, 1995).

For these theorists, spiritual growth occurs through stages which are sequential and hierarchical. In general, the lower stages focus on fulfillment of basic needs and ego development followed by ego disintegration with the recognition of ego insufficiency, and then movement to the higher stages involving an awareness of, acceptance of, and cooperation with transcendent forces. Movement through these stages reflects qualitative changes in one's view of the world and in all relationships. The process of spiritual growth is becoming connected with self, others, and God or the transcendent. Spiritual growth reduces dysfunctioning, enhances maximum functioning, and is inextricably linked to growth in the bio-psycho-social dimensions.

Movement from one stage to the next occurs through a death-rebirth transformative process. This change in the person as a result of breaking away from the past may be described as transcendence, which Ellison (1983) defines as "a stepping back from and moving beyond what is" (p. 331). From this definition, transcendence would include (1) moving developmentally from one stage to the next through the lower stages as well as into and through the higher stages and (2) moving beyond the individual self (as defined at a particular time) as well as beyond all human selves into a full realization of the cosmic reality. Depending on one's stage, experiential and conscious awareness of the transcendent as a separate aspect may or may not be present.

Many hold that spiritual or personality growth through these stages occurs within the context of one's life experiences, either predictable developmental crises or unpredictable and/or traumatic events (Canda, 1988c; Carroll, 1997a; Jaffe, 1985). Stressful or traumatic events (e.g., war, life-threatening illnesses) may initially impede growth. Similarly, the effects of abuse during childhood as well as unhealthy and dysfunctional adult behaviors (including addictions) may also delay growth as the behaviors reflect part(s) of oneself which is/are disconnected from self. The disconnected part(s) need(s) to be acknowledged and owned.

As the stressful experiences are or become perceived as a challenge, the person becomes unstuck and resumes growing (Golan, 1978). This perception has the potential for placing such behaviors in a larger perspective so that rather than the person being in opposition to God or the transcendent, one's behaviors become a way through which one's lack of connectedness (with self, others, and/or God) may be addressed and one's potential may emerge. This view is reflected in some recovering alcoholics gratefully remarking that without the alcoholism, "I wouldn't be where I am today" (Carroll, 1997a; Netting & Thibault, 1999) and supports the belief that one of the clinician-client tasks is to discover meanings through which suffering is transformed into growth opportunity (Canda & Furman, 1999).

Persons who have made transformational changes following trauma, stress, or psychological problems have participated in a creative restructuring of the self. They have been curious and involved in whatever is happening, and have been challenged by changes which stimulated healing and growth. These events and experiences represent tests for the psyche. They become opportunities for self renewal, growth, and transformation by assisting and motivating persons to wonder about their origins and identities as well as to search for life's purpose and for some transcendent meaning (Carroll, 1999; Jaffe, 1985).

A WHOLISTIC MODEL

Limitations of Current Diagrammatic Models

The diagrammatic models reviewed here that depict human nature and the place of spirituality in it have several limitations. First, these current models seem to have a closed quality in that only the Vertical-Horizontal Approach is diagrammed in a way so as to show growth. The diagrams do not provide a way to illustrate where someone is in the various dimensions at one point in time and thereby to chart the development of spirituality (defined as the transpersonal dimension and as a person's essence) over time.

Second, these models do not address either the origin or the beginning of spirituality. For instance, how does one's spirituality, a person's very being, fit into the ultimate reality? Can spirituality be absent? It has sometimes been described as nonexistent. This description seems reasonable particularly when spirituality is defined quantitatively as in the transpersonal (vertical) dimension of the Vertical-Horizontal Model. A zero point would indicate that no conscious relationship (with God or the transcendent) exists and that the amount or level of the existing relationship theoretically can be measured. This model also includes the possibility of minus zero "scores" which would thus frame the vertical dimension in terms of the quality (positive or negative) of the relationship. With respect to spirituality as one's core nature, its nonexistence seems impossible. How can spirituality not exist since, without the spirit (defined as core or essence), humans are physically not even alive? And there is much evidence that people who lose faith and hope physically die.

And third, the existing models do not account for references in the literature to negative and/or distorted images of the transcendent. For instance, many persons, especially those who struggle with addictions, believe in an all-judging, punitive God and frequently also have difficulties with experiencing a power greater than self, sharing self with others or hearing who they are (Carroll, 1997a), accepting self and others as imperfect (Kurtz & Ketcham, 1992), and living without fear and resentment (Dollard in Prugh, 1985/1986).

A New Model

This writer suggests a new model, Spirituality: A Wholistic Model, which includes aspects of earlier models (core essence, relationship with God or the transpersonal, and manifestations of that relationship) (see Figure 7). It acknowledges an open-endedness to spiritual development and provides a way of charting developmental growth. Similar to other models with vertical and horizontal axes, the horizontal axis reflects relationship with self, others, and

FIGURE 7. Spirituality: A Wholistic Model. Constructed by author.

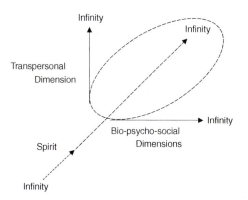

the world while the vertical axis reflects relationship with the transcendent (which may or may not be according to traditional organized religious beliefs). In contrast, the two axes do not intersect or meet. This lack of a meeting point allows space for spirit to enter thus indicating the beginning of human life and placing one's being in a larger context. The axes explicitly do not end as they move outward into infinity. The total space between the two axes, noted here by the open circle (but may be another shape), is where growth occurs. The circle does not have rigid boundaries but represents possibilities of growth and expansion upward and outward. This diagram provides a way to see the relationship between the transpersonal dimension and the bio-psycho-social dimensions, *all* of which are grounded within a universal spiritual context (similar to Absolute Spirit in Five Levels of Consciousness).

According to this model, manifestations of a person's experiences and relationships with self and others would be at a specific developmental stage on the bio-psycho-social axis. The degree of his or her relationship with God or a Higher Power (however conceptualized) would be indicated on the transpersonal axis. The boundaries of their interconnection, at any one time, would form a circle or some other shape.

In describing spirituality, people frequently use positive terms, such as fulfilling, meaningful, and peaceful. For this reason, the term, "negative spirituality" (reflected in a below zero rating in the Vertical-Horizontal approach) is somewhat confusing. One way of understanding the descriptions identified as negative spirituality is through the relationship between the bio-psycho-social and the transpersonal dimensions. A person may see his or her negative beliefs about self, others, and human relationships as negative aspects of God or the transcendent. In other words, the negative beliefs (which may well reflect one's human relationships and experiences) may be projected on to the transcendent. In this situation, a person having these "negative" beliefs would be low on the transpersonal axis (little relationship with the transcendent) and would be at a specific developmental level on the bio-psycho-social axis. Then, the characteristics of "negative spirituality" might be attributed to the effects of traumatic or other problematic events and experiences.

The difference between the transpersonal dimension and spirituality presents another way of understanding "negative spirituality." For instance, some religions believe in a conditional God who is judgmental or negative and is not "all-loving." This belief seems to refer to an image of God (or a negative view of the transcendent) rather than to spirituality, which is generally considered to be a life-giving principle or force.

CONCLUSION

The importance of social work practice and spirituality has been increasingly recognized. Recent books (Bullis, 1996; Canda & Furman, 1999; Robbins, Chatterjee, & Canda, 1998) explore a variety of ways, such as transpersonal theories, strengths perspective, multicultural approaches, and growth-oriented helping techniques, which are important to understanding spirituality within this profession.

All-too-often, theoretical frameworks or practice interventions are emphasized one over the other, yet the two are inextricably intertwined. Conceptual models are designed to (and do) enhance our understanding of the integration of theory and practice, but the conceptualizations themselves can be difficult to follow. Diagrammatic models help to clarify concepts and to facilitate understanding of the theory-practice integration.

This new diagrammatic model, Spirituality: A Wholistic Model, provides a visual way of understanding and assessing the person-in-environment currently and of following changes over time. Grounded in a multi-dimensional theoretical foundation, this model provides a way to evaluate the helpfulness of experiences, including practice interventions, with respect to their role in assisting each individual in moving toward realization of full potential. Although the goal may not primarily be that of managed care, the positive relationship between spiritual growth and improved everyday psycho-social functioning (Carroll, 1997a, 1999; Smith, 1995) supports the compatibility of managed care and spiritual approaches.

This model also ties into the work of Canda and Furman (1999) by providing another way of connecting the conceptual underpinnings of their holistic and operational models of spirituality. Developing new ways to understand the whole person assists social workers in being more responsive to fully accepting clients, to meeting the needs of clients, and to providing services responsibly as we move into the 21st century.

REFERENCES

Berenson, D. (1987). Alcoholics Anonymous: From surrender to transformation. *Family Therapy Networker*, 11(4), 25-31.
Bullis, R. K. (1996). *Spirituality in social work practice*. Washington, DC: Taylor & Francis.
Canda, E. R. (1983). General implications of shamanism for clinical social work. *International Social Work*, 26(4), 14-22.
Canda, E. R. (1986). *A conceptualization of spirituality for social work: Its issues and implications.* Unpublished doctoral dissertation, Ohio State University, Columbus.
Canda, E. R. (1988a). Conceptualizing spirituality for social work: Insights from diverse perspectives. *Social Thought*, 14(1), 30-46.
Canda, E. R. (1988c). Therapeutic transformation in ritual, therapy, and human development. *Journal of Religion and Health*, 27(3), 205-220.
Canda, E. R. (1990). Afterword: Spirituality reexamined. *Spirituality and Social Work Communicator*, 1(1), 13-14.
Canda, E. R. (1997). Spirituality. In R. L. Edwards (Ed.-in-Chief), *Encyclopedia of social work* (19th ed., supplement, pp. 299-310). Washington, DC: NASW Press
Canda, E. R., & Furman, L. D. (1999). *Spiritual diversity in social work practice*. New York: The Free Press.
Carroll, M. M. (1997a). Spirituality, Alcoholism, and Recovery: An exploratory study. *Alcoholism Treatment Quarterly*, 15(4), 89-98.
Carroll, M. M. (1997b). Spirituality and clinical social work: Implications of past and current perspectives. *Arete*, 22(1), 25-34.
Carroll, M. M. (1998). Social work's conceptualization of spirituality. In Edward R. Canda (Ed.), *Spirituality in social work: New directions* (pp. 1-13). Binghamton, NY: The Haworth Pastoral Press.
Carroll, M. M. (1999). Spirituality and alcoholism: Self-actualization and faith stage. *Journal of Ministry in Addiction & Recovery*, 6(1), 67-84.
Carson, V. B. (1989a). Spiritual development across the life span. In V. Carson (Ed.), *Spiritual dimensions of nursing practice* (pp. 24-51). Philadelphia: W. B. Saunders.
Corbett, L. (1925). Spiritual factors in casework. *The Family*, VI(8), 223-227.
Cornett, C. (1992). Toward a more comprehensive personology: Integrating a spiritual perspective into social work practice. *Social Work*, 37(2), 101-102.
Cowley, A. S. (1993). Transpersonal social work: A theory for the 1990s. *Social Work*, 38(5), 527-534.
Dudley, J. R., & Helfgott, C. (1990). Exploring a place for spirituality in the social work curriculum. *Journal of Social Work Education*, 26(3), 287-294.
Ellison, C. W. (1983). Spiritual well-being: conceptualization and measurement. *Journal of Psychology and Theology*, 11(4), 330-340.

Ellor, J. W., Netting, F. E., & Thibault, J. M. (1999). *Understanding religious and spiritual aspects of human service practice.* Columbia, SC: University of South Carolina Press.

Farran, C. J., Fitchett, G., Quiring-Emblen, J. D., & Burck, J. R. (1989). Development of a model for spiritual assessment and intervention. *Journal of Religion and Health,* 28(3), 185-194.

Fowler, J. W. (1981). *Stages of faith.* New York: Harper & Row.

Golan, N. (1978). *Treatment in crisis situations.* New York: The Free Press.

Helminiak, D. A. (1987). *Spiritual development.* Chicago: Loyola University Press.

Jaffe, D. T. (1985). Self-renewal. *Journal of Humanistic Psychology,* 25(4), 99-124.

Joseph, M. V. (1988). Religion and social work practice. *Social Casework,* 69(7), 443-452.

Jung, C. G. (1933). *Modern man in search of a soul.* New York: Harcourt Brace Jovanovich.

Jung, C. G. (1954a). Development of personality. In *Collected works* (Vol. 17, pp. 167-186). Princeton, NJ: Princeton University Press. (Translated from "Wirklichkeit der Seele," *Wirklichkeit der Seele* 1934, Zurich: Rascher).

Keith-Lucas, A. (1960). Some notes on theology and social work. *Social Casework,* 41(2), 87-91.

Kilpatrick, A. C., & Holland, T. P. (1990). The spiritual dimensions of practice. *The Clinical Supervisor,* 8(2), 125-140.

Kurtz, E., & Ketcham, K. (1992). *The spirituality of imperfection.* New York: Bantam Books.

Maslow, A. (1962). *Toward a psychology of being.* New York: Van Nostrand.

Maslow, A. H. (1971). Self-Actualizing and beyond. In *Farther reaches of human nature* (pp. 41-56). New York: The Viking Press. (Reprinted from *Challenges of humanistic psychology,* by J. F. T. Bugental, Ed., 1967, New York: McGraw-Hill Company)

O'Brien, P. J. (1992). Social work and spirituality: Clarifying the concept for practice. *Spirituality and Social Work Journal,* 3(1), 2-5.

Ortiz, L. P. A. (1991). Religious issues: The missing link in social work education. *Spirituality and Social Work Communicator,* 2(2), 13-18.

Prugh, T. (1985/1986, Winter). Alcohol, spirituality, and recovery. *Alcohol, Health, and Research World,* 28-31, 53-4.

Richmond, M. (1930). *The Long View.* New York: Russell Sage Foundation.

Robbins, S., Chatterjee, P., & Canda, E. R. (1998). *Contemporary human behavior theory: A critical perspective for social work.* Boston: Allyn & Bacon.

Sermabeikian, P. (1994). Our clients, ourselves: The spiritual perspective and social work practice. *Social Work,* 39(2), 178-183.

Siporin, M. (1985). Current social work perspectives on clinical practice. *Clinical Social Work Journal,* 13(3), 198-217.

Smith, E. D. (1995). Addressing the psychospiritual distress of death as reality: A transpersonal approach. *Social Work,* 40, 402-412.

Stoll, R. I. (1989). The essence of spirituality. In V. Carson (Ed.). *Spiritual dimensions of nursing practice* (pp. 4-23). Philadelphia: W. B. Saunders.

Titone, A. M. (1991). Spirituality and psychotherapy in social work practice. *Spirituality and Social Work Communicator*, 2(1), 7-9.

Vaughan, F. E. (1985, 1995). *The inward arc: Healing in psychotherapy and spirituality* (2nd ed.). Nevada City, CA: Blue Dolphin Publishing.

Washburn, M. (1995). *The ego and the dynamic ground* (2nd ed.). Albany, NY: State University New York.

Weick, A. (1983b). Issues in overturning a medical model of social work practice. *Social Work*, 28(6), 467-471.

Wilber, K., Engler, J., & Brown, D. P. (1986). *Transformations of consciousness*. Boston: New Science Library/Shambhala.

Transpersonal Psychology and Deep Ecological Philosophy: Exploring Linkages and Applications for Social Work

Fred H. Besthorn

SUMMARY. This article broadens the way social work understands the ways humanity defines and shapes its individual and collective realities in relation to nature. It incorporates and links relevant knowledge from transpersonal psychology and deep ecological philosophy in an effort to formulate fresh avenues for defining, pursuing, and resolving the many challenges that humankind faces at the dawn of this new millenium. The article concludes by suggesting some points of connection for generating a trans/ecological approach to social work and how this may portend important shifts of focus in social work theory and practice. *[Article copies available for a fee from The Haworth Document Delivery Service: 1-800-342-9678. E-mail address: <getinfo@haworthpressinc.com> Website: <http://www.HaworthPress.com> © 2001 by The Haworth Press, Inc. All rights reserved.]*

KEYWORDS. Transpersonal, deep ecology, spirituality, social work, environment

---

Fred H. Besthorn, PhD, is Assistant Professor in the Department of Social Work at Washburn University, 1700 College Avenue, Topeka, KS 66621 (E-mail: zzbest@washburn.edu).

[Haworth co-indexing entry note]: "Transpersonal Psychology and Deep Ecological Philosophy: Exploring Linkages and Applications for Social Work." Besthorn, Fred H. Co-published simultaneously in *Social Thought* (The Haworth Press, Inc.) Vol. 20, No. 1/2, 2001, pp. 23-44; and: *Transpersonal Perspectives on Spirituality in Social Work* (ed: Edward R. Canda, and Elizabeth D. Smith) The Haworth Press, Inc. 2001, pp. 23-44. Single or multiple copies of this article are available for a fee from The Haworth Document Delivery Service [1-800-342-9678, 9:00 a.m. - 5:00 p.m. (EST). E-mail address: getinfo@haworthpressinc.com].

INTRODUCTION

For much of the last quarter century, the social work profession has encountered a growing array of alternative conceptual approaches, from various points on the intellectual spectrum, which have competed with the profession's conventional theoretical models of human development. For example, in recent years we have seen a small but growing body of postmodern social critique challenging the reductionist, materialistic, and hierarchical assumptions of the positivist/empiricist world view (Imre, 1982; Roberts, 1990; Saleebey, 1991, 1996; Weick, 1981, 1991), as well as alternative viewpoints delineating the relevance and application to social work of such theoretical constructs as strengths-based perspectives (De Jong & Miller, 1995; Saleebey, 1991, 1996), chaos/complexity theory (Warren, Franklin & Streeter, 1998), empowerment theory (Gutierrez, 1994; Gutierrez, DeLois & GlenMaye, 1995), spiritual beliefs and practices (Canda, 1989, 1991, 1997; Canda & Furman, 1999), constructionist and constructivist approaches (Fleck-Henderson, 1993; Granvold, 1996), and feminist perspectives (Van Den Berg, 1995).

Schriver (1998) reminds the profession that we have too often limited the integration of knowledge for conceptual development to the narrow confines of traditional sociological and behavioral scientific theory. In doing so the profession has failed to appreciate and utilize the full range of epistemological innovation that has occurred in the arts, humanities, philosophy, critical theory, and ecological/systems perspectives–to name but a few. This omission, or perhaps oversimplification, has not been without consequence for the profession. In Schriver's (1998) words, we have "cheated ourselves out of some of the most current, exciting, and challenging streams of thought" while most problematically "denying the people with and for whom we work important new avenues for defining, pursuing, and resolving many of the problems with which we must deal" (p. xiii).

Accordingly, this chapter will expand the profession's theoretical base for understanding the human condition and the course of human development. It aims to broaden professional awareness by incorporating and linking relevant knowledge from both transpersonal psychology and deep ecological philosophy. Transpersonal theory and deep ecology are by definition alternative paradigms. They represent new (in the sense of having had less influence and prominence in the Western academic tradition) perspectives on the way we define and shape ourselves within our individual and collective environments. Yet, much of their metaphysics are as ancient as antiquity, reflecting contemplative and wisdom traditions from a variety of past and contemporary cultures.

Transpersonal theory and deep ecology create exciting and largely un-tapped potentialities for perceiving ourselves, others, and the universe–both in and around us. They also present some special difficulties for professionals thoroughly steeped in Western social and professional value assumptions of individuality, self-mastery, rationality, and ego strength (Robbins, Chatterjee, & Canda, 1998). They require that we temporarily set aside some of our comfort-able presuppositions about the cosmos and instead embrace some degree of ambiguity while opening ourselves to ways of knowing and doing that reflect more holistic and trans-egoic perspectives.

TRANSPERSONAL PSYCHOLOGY

Historical Development

Transpersonal psychology represents a new institutional force in modern, western psychology. It has been called the *fourth force* of psychology because it challenges and moves beyond the theoretical influence of the first three in-stitutional movements: Freudianism, behaviorism, and humanistic psychol-ogy (Robbins, Chatterjee, & Canda, 1998). Humanistic psychology is the immediate theoretical predecessor of transpersonal psychology. It emerged in the 1950s and 1960s in response to the deterministic and rather pessimistic view of human nature espoused by both the behaviorist and Freudian schools. The primary impetus of the humanistic school was to focus on de-veloping those unique and positive components of the human psyche such as meaningfulness, creativity, and subjective experience as critical components to the formation of individual self-actualization (Okun, 1997; Robbins, Chatterjee, & Canda, 1998).

Abraham Maslow (1908-1970), an early progenitor of the humanistic move-ment, felt that behavorists had simply ignored the volitional, internality of the human organism; while focusing on the external, mechanistic nature of human activity. The Freudians, though recognizing the importance of the interior life, could only see one's interior consciousness as leading to some form of neurotic misery (Fox, 1995). Maslow asserted in his 1954 book, *Motivation and Person-ality,* that psychology had been more successful revealing humanity's shortcom-ings, illnesses, and sins rather than its potentialities, virtues, aspirations, or full psychological development. "It is as if psychology had voluntarily restricted it-self to only half its rightful jurisdiction, and that the darker, meaner half" (Maslow, 1954, p. 354). Traditional behavioralism and psycho-dynamic models had forgotten that the human psyche includes many good qualities, such as joy, rapture, laughter, simple daily happiness, and rare moments of ecstasy and self transcendence (Kaluger & Kaluger, 1984; Maslow, 1971).

As humanistic psychology became institutionalized in the turbulent and psychedelic milieu of the counter-cultural 1960s, it became apparent to some within the movement that the humanistic perspective was still not able to accommodate significant aspects of the human experience (Kaluger & Kaluger, 1984). The self that most humanistic psychologists were seeking to bring to actualization was not all that different from the self of psychoanalytic depth psychology. The self with which most humanistic psychologists were concerned still tended to be conceived as a skin-encapsulated ego, a separate "I"-ness (Fox, 1995).

Thus, beginning in the 1960s and 1970s, a new transpersonal psychology began to emerge, espousing an expanded theory of human consciousness. This new impetus sprang from insights within the humanistic perspective, but was also strongly influenced by three other streams of intellectual thought: existential philosophy, transpersonal psychodynamic theory, and the study of alternative states of consciousness (Cowley, 1993; Hutchison, 1999; Robbins, Chatterjee, & Canda, 1998). Many innovative thinkers have surfaced to develop the empirical and theoretical bases of transpersonal theory, including Stanislav Grof, Charles Tart, Frances Vaughan, Roger Walsh, Michael Washburn and Ken Wilber. Transpersonal psychology ascribes to a view of human consciousness which is far more expansive than conventional Western psychological notions. It views development as a process of continual transcendence where a sense of self evolves "that extends beyond one's egoic, biographical or personal sense of self" (Vaughn, 1980, p. 16).

Core Concepts

Transpersonal psychology's core concepts are difficult to categorize partly because they have developed from such a varied array of intellectual traditions, ranging from minority traditions in Western theology and psychology to Eastern spiritual practices (Cowley, 1993; Cowley & Derezotes, 1994; Fox, 1995; Robbins, Chatterjee, & Canda, 1998). However, transpersonal theory does have several unifying concepts. The first is related to the way the idea of expanded consciousness is defined. Transpersonal theorists share the belief that human experiences can and ought to be conceived of in ways that extend the view of consciousness beyond conventional ego boundaries and space/time constraints. That is, the individual should be understood as capable of identifying "with aspects of the world and humanity beyond the body, transcending the condition of separateness and isolation in recognition of the interrelated unity of existence" (Walsh, 1984, p. 459). From a transpersonal perspective, failure to appreciate that human beings are capable of realizing non-ordinary, mystical, spiritual states of consciousness is to leave the human psyche trapped in an egocentric confinement. Western therapeutic systems are consequently designed simply to "patch up" (Wilber, 1977, p. 20) suffering, the neurotic and sometimes psychotic manifestations of this confinement, rather than helping the self truly transcend its egoic limitations.

Transpersonal adherents see the absence of an appropriate vision of the transcending self as the source of both micro and macro level dysfunction. Speaking as a social work transpersonal practitioner, Cowley (1993) recognized that visions of reality "that do not recognize higher levels of consciousness may inhibit clients' development and also contribute to their misdiagnosis" (p. 530). For transpersonalists, higher consciousness is "the epitome of health and well-being," according to Cowley and Derezotes (1994, p. 34). At the macro level, transpersonalists such as social critic Willis Harman (1998) recognize that "since modern culture ascribes no 'reality' to inner experience" (p. 127), transcendent values have no power to inform us and, as a result, materialistic and egocentric values prevail. Thus, economic profit-based rationalization and self-gratification become an ever-increasing portion of individual behavior and social organization.

A second core concept of transpersonal psychology is related to the way it understands the developmental processes of individuals and the social order. Ken Wilber (1977, 1983, 1986, 1993, 1995, 1996, 1998), one of transpersonal psychology's most prolific writers and seminal theorists, concludes that human beings are the product of an evolutionary process that involves not only biology and culture but increasingly comprehensive levels of individual and collective spiritual sensibility and higher consciousness. Each new level integrates all previous levels and represents development toward a transpersonal level of awareness (Besthorn, 1997; Robbins, Chatterjee, & Canda, 1998).

For Wilber, the remedy for individual ego alienation and social inequity is not to find unity with a divine other, whether understood personally, ecologically, or celestially, but rather an enlightenment into an all-embracing, nondual, generative awareness (Besthorn, 1997; Zimmerman, 1994). Enlightenment recognizes that perceived separateness between things or dimensions of reality (persons/persons, person/God, person/nature, emotion/reason, spirit/body) is an illusion. Dualistic merger with anything other is problematic because it blinds the immersed to a deeper sense of the *over-soul* (Wilber, 1995, p. 288). The over-soul is a type of metaphysical quintessence which exists within but beyond the identifiable, sensory reality of person and culture. But, it is the essence out of which loving embrace of person, culture, and nature emerge (Besthorn, 1997). Wilber suggests that when a person or sociocultural system *remembers* its original connection with the Absolute, rather than seeking merger with the Absolute, it is freed from "the chains of alienation and separate-self existence" (Wilber, 1981, p. 12). This remembering "corresponds to a true mystical state, in which all boundaries and dualism have been transcended and all individuality dissolves into universal, undifferentiated oneness" (Capra, 1983, p. 371).

Wilber (1977) speculates that individuals and social environments share parallel developmental courses toward full spiritual enlightenment. He refers to this increasingly complex and sophisticated ordering of individual consciousness and social organization as the *spectrum of consciousness.* He utilizes the idea of holons as a descriptive metaphor for the systemic development of both individual and social processes (Wilber, 1995). For Wilber, the evolution of individual and social consciousness is holonic. It is a cyclical, upward spiraling of expanding complexity with various bands or circles (holons) that exhibit infinite shades and gradations, building upon, including, and transcending previous developmental levels. Each ascending level represents a more sophisticated and comprehensive mode of consciousness. It is not a linear progression through a series of stages as most conventional developmental theorists such as Piaget, Erikson, and Kohlberg have suggested.

A final core concept of transpersonal theory is related to how it views the progress of individual and social developmental schema. Most transpersonal theorists do not believe that progress to higher evolutionary states of consciousness are inevitable. Without a personal and social transformation of thought and action, the kind of evolutionary development conceived by transpersonalists will not come to fruition. Indeed, most transpersonalists would agree with social ecologist Murray Bookchin's (1986) observations that "we may well be approaching a crucial juncture in our development that confronts us with a historic choice: whether we will follow an alternative path that yields a human, rational, and ecological way of life, or a path which will yield the degradation of our species, if not its outright extinction" (p. 99).

From a transpersonal perspective, social conditions and personal actions are the outward expression of inward sentiments. All problems are deeply interconnected. Thus nothing will change significantly unless everything changes. As Wilber (1986) described it:

> at this point in history, the most radical, earth shaking transformation would occur simply if everyone truly evolved to a mature rational, and responsible ego capable of freely participating in the open exchange of mutual self-esteem. There is the edge of history. There would be a real new age. (p. 328)

A central issue for many transpersonal theorists is that every transformation to a higher level of consciousness carries with it a *regressive temptation* for individuals or societies to move backwards, developmentally, in order to re-inhabit forms of life that they have outgrown but which seem more preferable to present uncertainty and discomfort (diZerega, 1996). This predilection towards regression portends significant problems for society. It carries a *repressive tendency* to suppress anyone extolling change in a forward-looking direction or anyone not willing to adopt the myth of perpetual stability and temporal immortality. The aesthetic penchant and vocal calls for a nationalistic moral agenda of prewar German Nazism is sometimes cited as the most virulent expression of society seeking to ward off the discomfort of change. Wilber (1986, 1995) refers to this as a form of the *pre-trans fallacy* because of the common impulse of individuals and societies to confuse *pre*personal levels of development with *trans*personal levels. For transpersonal theorists, their most important task is to contribute to a transformative, forward-looking change in the consciousness of Western society. They would find agreement with the conviction that by "changing their images of reality, people are changing the world" (Harman, 1998, p. xviii).

DEEP ECOLOGY

Historical Development

According to Devall and Sessions (1985), the term deep ecology was coined by the Norwegian philosopher Arne Naess in his 1973 article *The Shallow and the Deep, Long Range Ecology Movements*. In this article Naess attempted to describe a deeper and more experientially grounded approach to human development by explicating the important connection between human and natural ecological systems. He offers a distinction between a shallow and a deep ecology movement. Shallow ecology is concerned with ecological problems because of their impact on humans in the industrialized world. Deep ecology is more deeply concerned with issues of ecological equality in humanity's fundamental relationship with nature. Many theorists have been expanding Naess' original conceptualizations in an attempt to provide a thorough grounding for a new experiential philosophy of nature (e.g., Devall & Sessions, 1985; Drengson, 1995; Drengson & Inoue, 1995; Fox, 1990, 1995; LaChapelle, 1995; List, 1993; Macy, 1995; McLaughlin, 1993, 1995; Naess, 1984, 1988, 1989; Rothenberg, 1993; Sessions, 1992, 1995).

Merchant (1992) has noted a large number of religious, philosophical, and scientific influences on deep ecology. These include: (a) alternative western religious traditions, particularly that of Saint Francis of Assisi and the early modern transcendental movement, particularly the works of Emerson and

Thoreau; (b) eastern philosophy, such as that described by Daisetz Suzuki; (c) eastern religious traditions, for instance Taoism, Buddhism, Zen Buddhism, Hinduism, and the works of Mohandas Gandhi; (d) First Nations traditions from such teachers as Black Elk and Luther Standing Bear; (e) alternative western philosophy represented in the works of Giordano Bruno, Gottfried Leibniz, Baruch Spinoza, and George Santayana; (f) radical scientific critiques of modern ecology, particularly the work of Paul Shepard; (g) radical sociological and philosophical critique of the dominant western worldview in the work of William Catton, Riley Dunlap, and Martin Heidegger; (h) the new physics represented in the work of Fritjof Capra; and (i) the new systemic challenge to the mechanistic model of nature predicated upon the holistic, self-organizing character of systems and represented in the achievements of David Bohm, Ilya Prigogine, Edward Lorenz, Charles Birch, and James Lovelock.

Sessions (1995a) suggests that the evolution of deep ecology was also influenced by the *political activism* of the 1960s, particularly that of the so-called Environmental Revolution. Both grew out of the newly emerging science of ecology and an often unconscious sense related not only to protecting nature but to developing a closer relationship with it. This need to reconnect with nature was popularized in Aldo Leopold's (1949) ethics of the land and Rachel Carson's (1962) pivotal book, *Silent Spring* (Sessions, 1995a). Carson's book dealt specifically with the use of pesticides and their impact on small animal life, but her ultimate concerns went far deeper to critique the direction and goals of western society to dominate nature (Sessions, 1995b).

Core Concepts

Drengson and Inoue (1995, p. xxi) make the point that the term "deep ecology" has two general connotations. One refers to a broad ecocentric grassroots movement to achieve an ecologically balanced future. The other is reserved for the "specific ecological philosophy" of Arne Naess, and other theorists who have expanded upon his original thought. While admitting the difficulty in separating the movement from its philosophy, Drengson and Inoue suggest that the term *deep ecology* be used to refer to the philosophy while the phrase *deep ecology movement* be used when referring to the grassroots movement. In either case, deep ecology attempts to articulate a long-range ecological vision that reflects a deeper connection and openness between humans and between humans and the non-human world while doing what is required to protect ecocentric values and the integrity of the earth's ecological communities.

There are a number of core concepts of deep ecological thought which act to consolidate the beliefs of many who identify themselves as deep ecologists. The first is related to the idea of an *expanded sense of self consciousness*. Fox

(1984) argued the "central intuition" of deep ecology is that there is no onto-logical divide in the field of existence. That is, the world is not divided into subjects and objects nor is there any separation in reality between the human and nonhuman realm. Rather "all entities are constituted by their relationships. To the extent that we perceive boundaries, we fall short of a deep ecological consciousness" (p. 196). McLaughlin (1987, p. 2) suggested that the heart of deep ecology is the cultivation of "ecological consciousness" by which he meant deep ecology's insistence upon bringing to the forefront the question of how should I be rather than addressing abstract and dispassionate questions about the essence of value and the structure of moral argument. McLaughlin (1995) added that deep ecology's heart—expansion of self toward ecological consciousness—is the primary basis for "rejecting consumerism" which creates and sustains "the loss of traditional ways of forming one's identity and their re-placement by material possessions" (p. 263).

In his 1973 article, Naess (cited in List, 1993, p. 19) suggested that cultivat-ing ecological consciousness involves moving away from a view of per-son-in-environment to one of self as part of a "relational total-field." That is, rather than experiencing ourselves as separate from our environment and exist-ing *in* it, we begin to cultivate the insight that we are *with* our environment. Be-ing *with* environment means appreciating that we are part of a complex totality of interconnected relationships and that these connections with human and non-human others is the very essence of our self-identity.

Naess understands this sense of self in terms of the process of identification and alienation. That is, one's self is that with which one identifies, and not-self is that from which one is alienated. If one thinks of this fluctuating sense of self as a continuum, self-realization at its maximum is identification in its widest sense, a oneness in diversity (diversity here extended to all beings in the uni-verse) while a limited egoistic self-realization is a maximum of alienation and a narrow, constricted sense of what constitutes one's self (Naess, 1989). Naess (1988) distinguished between his concept of maximum self-realization and the one commonly used in modern society to mean the "competitive develop-ment of a person's talents and the pursuit of an individual's specific inter-ests" (p. 263). From this latter view an inherent conflict is seen between developing a sense of individual self and cultivating bonds with significant others, family, community, and, as importantly, extending to nature.

This conflict reflects Western social theory's typical dualistic, egoism-altruism distinction. According to this view, altruism (selfless care for others) is a moral quality developed by suppression of selfishness in favor of others. Naess challenges this thinking by proposing that one can cultivate con-nections with others, with family, and with nature without losing some part of self. He contends that maximum self-realization arises only in the context of maximum diversity "by an increase in the number of ways in which individuals, societies, and even species and life forms realize themselves" (Bodian, 1995, p. 30).

As one develops ever-widening identification, there is no need for a self-sacrificing, moral altruism since the interests of those with whom we identify, nature included, may be seen as one's own interests as well. Self becomes most fully realized not solely when self-interest and wants are met, but rather when one begins to identify with more than one's own self. By reframing the developmental process in this way, deep ecology challenges shallow theories of self differentiation and the inherent conflicts arising from competing needs among isolated egos. Maturing involves a process of widening one's sense of self and identifying with others–family, friends, communities, our own species, and then all species of non-human life.

Deep questioning is a second core theme of deep ecology. For deep ecologists, cultivating a total view of human/human and particularly human/nonhuman relationships necessarily requires engagement in a process of deep questioning. In a 1982 interview, Naess argued:

> The essence of deep ecology is to ask deeper questions . . . ecology as a science does not ask what kind of a society would be the best for maintaining a particular ecosystem–that is considered a question for value theory, for politics, for ethics. As long as ecologists keep narrowly to their science, they do not ask such questions. . . . in deep ecology . . . we question our society's underlying assumptions. . . . We are not limited to a scientific approach; we have an obligation to verbalize a total view. . . . In general, however, people do not question deeply enough to explicate . . . a total view. (Devall & Sessions, 1985, p. 74)

Naess makes clear that deep ecology's approach to a broad range of environmental and social issues involves integrating one's intuitive capacities for person/other relationships and manifesting these by questioning "deeply and publicly, insistently and consistently" (Naess, 1995c, p. 75) the societal paradigm within which burdensome social and environmental problems reside. In taking such an approach Naess insists upon fundamental individual and social change. But he rejects the problem-solving change approaches of shallow environmentalists and social reformers as stop-gap solutions which ultimately fail at the task of long-term transformation. Naess rejects the person-in-environment image with an epistemological activism which deeply questions the knowledge and institutions which maintain an abstract, overly intellectualized, and scientifically derived social and environmental structure.

The third core theme of deep ecology which helps define the deep ecology worldview is that of *biocentric equality* (Devall & Sessions, 1985; Naess, 1995a, 1995b, 1995d). Biocentric equality holds that all beings in the ecosphere have intrinsic value and have an equal right to flourish, grow, and reach their individual self-realization within the greater holistic self-realization (Naess, 1988). Biocentric equality views natural entities as independent of their perceived usefulness for human purposes. It suggests that humans should live in ways which have minimum impact on the rest of nature and that humanity's role is one of "plain citizen" (Devall & Sessions, 1985, p. 68) rather than "master-slave" (Naess, 1995e, p. 4). The latter power-coercive role is associated with social oppression as well as human oppression of and alienation from nature.

Biocentric equality underscores one of the most significant assumptions of deep ecology, the intrinsic worth of all living things. From this value flows deep ecology's non-anthropocentrism, tolerance of different views and orientations, open communication with persons and nature, the inclusion of animals and plants in the community, and intensified preservation and conservation efforts (Naess, 1995c). Intrinsic worth upholds the qualities of richness, complexity, diversity, and symbiosis in the evolutionary cycle. "It involves a re-visioning of life and evolution, changing from understanding evolution as 'progress' from 'lower' to 'higher' forms to understanding evolution as a magnificent expression of a multitude of forms of life" (McLaughlin, 1995, p. 87). Naess (1995e, p. 4) said that the principle is a "deep seated respect, or even veneration" for all ways and forms of life. It depends in part upon the deep pleasure and satisfaction humans receive from close partnership with other forms of life. But to restrict this to humans only is an anthropocentric bias which has detrimental effects upon the life quality of human and nonhuman existence.

LINKAGES BETWEEN TRANSPERSONAL THEORY AND DEEP ECOLOGY

Deep ecological and transpersonal models share a reliance on similar theoretical and historical traditions for their own unique perspectives on the course of human development. While there has been disagreement between the two camps on particular components of each framework (diZerega, 1996; Fox, 1995; Rothberg & Kelly; 1998; Wilber, 1995, 1996, 1998; Zimmerman, 1990, 1994, 1998), it is clear that both are posing profound and more spiritual or transcendent levels of human evolution than have been advanced by conventional development models used commonly in social work. The current section will address some of the linkages between deep ecology and transpersonal psychology.

First, both recognize an imperative for the emergence of a new paradigm of human progress. At the heart of this call for a new paradigm is the mutual aversion both have for particular epistemological and ontological pitfalls of the modern era. While acknowledging that modernity has had certain positive and emancipatory impacts on individual and cultural development, many transpersonalists and deep ecologists find modernity's focus on a dualistic, mechanistic and materialistic reality as having created a predominant world view nearly devoid of spiritual, feminist, transpersonal, and ecological values.

Wilber (1998, p. 298) suggested that the "disaster of modernity" is that it forgot the transcendental core of both consciousness and the natural environment. "Thus, it tended to dissociate mind and nature," leading to an ontological rift between nature as object and self as subject. Transpersonalists and deep ecologists contend that the downside of the modernist project that began with European rational Enlightenment was its creation of a subtle reductionism that compressed the world into that which could be described only in empirical terms. This fashioned a reality which "had no depth, no gradations, no interiors, no qualitative distinctions, but instead could be approached through an objectifying empiricist gaze" (Wilber, 1995, p. 132).

Transpersonalist Roger Walsh (1998) also suggested that the great problem with the modernist worldview is that it drew humanity's attention away from the vertical/transcendent capacities of humans toward the horizontal/temporal. He suggested that "with the denial of the possibility of developmental ascent, attention turned downward to the world. Instead of an infinite above, there was now a horizontal, infinite ahead" (Walsh, 1998, pp. 46-47). The universe became a kind of ontological flatland. Drengson (1995) critiqued the technocratic paradigm of modernism. Its shortcoming is its predisposition to "objectify persons and nonhuman nature. Intersubjective experience cannot be 'captured' or characterized in these terms. It becomes subjective in the pejorative sense, unreal, unimportant, irrelevant" (p. 82).

A second linkage between transpersonalists and deep ecologists is their belief that an expanded sense of self must emerge that is united with a larger cosmic purpose. While the terminology and understanding for this *consciousness-beyond* (Fox, 1995; Zimmerman, 1998) vary among the two movements, there is also a great deal of convergence on this core concept. Deep ecologist George Sessions maintained that deep ecology is a spiritual movement involving "the growth or increasing maturity of the self" (cited in Zimmerman, 1994, p. 83). This growth of self, what Naess (1989) calls *self-realization,* manifests itself in experiences of identification with other humans, non-human species, and natural ecosystems. For deep ecology, experientiality is less a matter of mystical or regressive reunification with nature than it is a kind of effortless, practical involvement in nature's everyday realities. Deep ecologists are relatively critical of national parks and wilderness areas for tending to make people spectators of nature rather than inviting them to be with it–to experience it (Turner, 1995). From Arne Naess' (1989) perspective "to 'only look at' nature is an extremely peculiar behavior. Experiencing an environment happens by doing something in it, by living in it, meditating and acting" (p. 63).

Transpersonal theory's language of the consciousness-beyond tends to focus on the discipline and practice necessary to fully experience transformed awareness. Transpersonal theorists (Murphy, 1998; Rothberg, 1998; Vaughn, 1995; Walsh, 1998; Walsh & Vaughan, 1980; Wilber, 1995) indicate that expanded consciousness, while potentially available to any who may wish to continue their growth and development, also involves rigorous practice to realize this transpersonal level. As Walsh (1998) counseled, consciousness transformation "requires a rigorous, authentic contemplative discipline" (p. 50). Wilber's (1998) description of the stages of spiritual unfolding, particularly the difference between peak and plateau spiritual experiences, unequivocally suggests that individual development toward transpersonal levels, though available to everyone to *pass through,* will only be mastered by relatively few. He writes:

> Whereas peak experiences can, and usually do, come spontaneously, in order to sustain them and turn them from a peak into a plateau–from a brief altered state into a more enduring trait–prolonged practice is required. . . . I know of few bona fide cases of plateau experiences that did not involve years of sustained spiritual practice. (p. 180)

The coalescence between deep ecological and transpersonal theory on this idea of a transformative expansion of self is becoming increasingly evident. Deep ecologist Warwick Fox (1995) has suggested that deep ecology's view of expanded self, because of its inherent psychological nature, would lead one to conclude that a better descriptor for the philosophy would be *transpersonal ecology.* He suggested that since expanded self:

> involves the realization of a sense of self that extends beyond (or that is trans-) one's egoic, biographical, or personal sense of self, the clearest, most accurate, and most informative term for this sense of deep ecology is, in my view, transpersonal ecology. (p. 197)

Both deep ecologists and transpersonalists support the conclusion that personal transformation should be concomitant with cultural and institutional change. They would agree that the temporal settings and circumstances that humans find themselves living with are clearly associated with conditions of consciousness. But altering the first without altering the latter is inconceivable. This is the third point of linkage between deep ecology and transpersonal theory: Psychological transformation must accompany sociopolitical change.

For deep ecologists, internal transformation is inseparable from an ecologically harmonious and sustainable society that values human and nonhuman diversity. This has widespread implications, particularly in the West, for political, economic, social, educational, welfare, and cultural systems. Echoing the importance of a broad based social agenda, Naess (1995f) contended that supporters of the deep ecology movement:

> do not consider the ecological crisis to be the only global crisis; there are also crises of social justice, and of war and organized violence . . . and . . . political problems which are only distantly related to ecology. (p. 453)

In a similar manner, deep ecologist McLaughlin (1995) contended that the sociopolitical focus of deep ecology is toward a radical ecocentrism. "Radical ecocentrism intends fundamental changes both in consciousness of industrial peoples and the economic structure of industrial society" (p. 270).

The psychological transformation envisioned by many transpersonalists and the attendant alteration of larger structural systems, while at times less explicit than the deep ecological approach, nonetheless affirms the relationship between internal and external transformation. Wilber suggested that "the single greatest world transformation would simply be the embrace of global reasonableness and pluralistic tolerance" (cited in Zimmerman, 1998, p. 190). In even stronger language, Wilber (1998) advanced a macro expression of transpersonal development processes by suggesting that a transformative spirituality of the kind he envisions:

> does not seek to bolster or legitimate any present worldview at all, but rather to provide true authenticity by shattering what the world takes as legitimate. Transformative spirituality, authentic spirituality, is therefore revolutionary. It does not legitimate the world, it breaks the world; it does not console the world, it shatters it. And it does not render the world content, it renders it undone. (p. 143)

Transpersonalist Frances Vaughn (1995) also suggested that transpersonal therapies aim to actively facilitate a process of both personal and social empowerment. From Vaughan's perspective, personal change has its concomitant in social change–that which she calls social empowerment. Although people may often feel afraid of taking responsibility for initiating change and sometimes feel overwhelmed by what they believe they cannot change, "a person who has a connection to the inner life of the soul can find a source of strength that does not give up hope of change" (p. 158).

DEFINING A TRANS/ECOLOGICAL SOCIAL WORK

There have been increasing numbers of social workers, utilizing various components of transpersonal and deep ecological theory, who advocate for their inclusion into social work theory and practice (Berger & Kelly, 1993; Besthorn, 1997, 1999, 2000; Besthorn & Canda, in press; Besthorn & Tegtmeier, 1999; Canda, 1989, 1991, 1996; Canda & Furman, 1999; Coates, 1999; Coates & McCay, 1995; Cowley, 1993, 1996; Cowley & Derezotes, 1994; Derezotes & Evans, 1995; Hoff & McNutt, 1994; Hoff & Polack, 1993; Hutchison, 1999; Park, 1996; Robbins, Chatterjee, & Canda, 1998; Russel, 1998; Smith & Gray, 1995). This last section joins with these previous works by suggesting a point of connection for a new *trans/ecological* social work perspective.

A trans/ecological perspective recognizes the need for a significant shift of focus in social work theory and practice. Conventional notions of human development in social work that focus on an isolated, temporally bound self that is alienated from higher consciousness and sensate expression with nature are no longer tenable perspectives for helping professions in these complex and uncertain times. A trans/ecological view of development posits that the self has much richer psychological, emotional, transcendent, and ecological potentialities. Social trends of transformation indicate that human beings are capable of and ready to explore wider levels of maturational development. Many social work practitioners are discovering that people are increasingly experiencing what Cowley (1993, p. 528) called the "postmodern malady." They are no longer satisfied in defining their lives by the mere skin-encapsulated boundary of their egoic personage, their abstract rationality, or by the pointless material acquisition of consumer products.

Recognizing the potential for extended human developmental capacity means significantly more than just adding another conceptual perspective to social work's long list of theories interpreting the human condition. It challenges the very core of assumptions and distinctions that have principally shaped the social work agenda. For the most part, the dominant Western worldview has rejected the language of self-transcendence and experiential connection with nature. It has been especially suspicious of attempts to articulate a trans-rational relationship between a reanimated nature and a resacralized humanity. Social work is in large measure a professional reflection of this mind set. It has gradually grown suspicious of knowledge and experience which cannot be fully quantified or rationally derived. It has endeavored to free itself from the so-called imprecision and irrationality of spirituality in order to strengthen its claim to full membership in the professional and academic communities. The result is a professional ethos that tends to distrust the language of higher transcendence, mystical connection, intuitive grasp. It has replaced this with a reverence for numbers and mechanistic metaphors.

A trans/ecological perspective is consistent with counter-trends in social work of the past 10 years that seek holistic and spiritually sensitive ways of thinking and practicing. It suggests that social work should not ignore how it has often unwittingly cooperated in creating a disenchanted world and desacralized humanity characterized by a mostly synthetic, spiritually muted, alienated feeling and lifestyle. It clearly identifies the modern proclivity to divorce humans from nature as contributing to a broad range of individual and social problems, including emotional, familial, economic, and class issues as well as mounting ecological crisis.

At the level of individual intervention, a trans/ecological perspective provides professional social workers with a meta-framework by which they can assist their clients in finding expression for the pain and loss due to human/nature split. Social worker John Coates (1999) suggested that as people in western society increasingly realize that self-absorbed consumption, through resource exploitation and ecosystem degradation, can never satisfy the deepest human need for belonging, "personal depression" and a collective "darkness of soul" will be the inevitable result. A trans/ecological perspective can provide a normative framework to help clients find "a new sense of purpose, meaning and connection in their lives" (Coates, 1999, p. 19). The anguish of the current situation can be part of a general awakening to a new level of consciousness, new ways of healing personal and social issues, and a new way of being with oneself, others, and the world around us.

Wilderness practice is one example of an applied trans/ecological perspective. It offers the opportunity to expand social workers' conceptual bases and practice strategies to help clients identify a more fully developed sense of consciousness (Besthorn & Tegtmeier, 1999). Wilderness practice can be understood as experiences with wild and pristine places as well as simple encounters with meadows, parks, plants, gardens, pets, domesticated and non-domesticated animals, and vegetated streetscapes in either rural or urban contexts. It encourages professionals and their clients to utilize the experiential, imaginative, and transpersonal properties of nature to realize a deeper sense of self. From the practitioner's perspective, reconnecting with nature undercuts the dualistic categories of client-expert and mind-body. It also challenges conventional practice wisdom that restricts helping to a fifty-minute hour within the confines of an agency or office. Its focus is not on analysis, interpretation or advice from social workers. Rather, it offers opportunities for profound human/nature encounters through which a transformative self can begin to emerge.

Children and adolescents may especially benefit from wilderness practice. Wilderness practice does not necessarily require busing large groups of children to the High Sierras. It can be as simple as bringing the natural environment to children through the introduction of household pets, horticultural interests, or a simple walk through a local park. The critical issue is not necessarily location, but rather facilitating empathetic capacities, fostering personal and collective responsibility, and building inner confidence and relation skills. Caring and playful interaction with small animals, tending flowers or gardens, or deeply connecting with urban green spaces can foster spiritual, intuitive and political sensitivities (Besthorn, 2000).

Even the largest urban environment has natural settings which can be visited, often within short driving distance. For instance, introducing a group of children to the natural world experienced daily on a small farm can be an exciting, moving, and soul altering experience. Touching, with eyes tightly closed the soft, the velvety nose of the cow; listening to the mother sow gently nursing her piglets; burying one's hands and face into the warm, wooly coat of the sheep; observing the undeniable bond between the mother horse and her wobbly new colt; gazing into a night sky full of a million stars unhindered by city lights–all of these are simple, yet meaningful encounters which can profoundly alter anyone's perspective on life, young or old (Besthorn, 1997; Besthorn & Canda, in press).

As the world grows ever more turbulent and uncertain and as it continues to shift toward a different mode of collective understanding and social organization, the profession of social work must also adjust. This new millennium will bring new, perhaps unprecedented, demands and opportunities. Whether the profession is prepared to meet these depends in large measure on the flexibility, innovation, and explanatory power of its theoretical frameworks to guide its tasks. The trans/ecological perspective is a way to begin the task of preparing ourselves for this future.

REFERENCES

Berger, R., & Kelly, J. (1993). Social work in the ecological crisis. *Social Work, 38*(5), 521-526.

Besthorn, F. H. (1997). *Reconceptualizing social work's person-in-environment perspective: Explorations in radical environmental thought.* Unpublished doctoral dissertation, University of Kansas, Lawrence.

Besthorn, F. H. (1999, June). *The spiritual dimensions of deep ecology and social work practice.* Paper presented at the national conference of the Society for Spirituality and Social Work, St. Louis, MO.

Besthorn, F. H. (2000, February). *Radical environmentalism: Reflections of educating social workers in spirituality and social justice.* Juried paper presented at the Annual Program Meeting of the Council on Social Work Education, New York, NY.

Besthorn, F. H., & Canda, E. R. (in press). Revisioning environment: Deep ecology for social work education. *Journal of Teaching in Social Work.*

Besthorn, F. H., & Tegtmeier, D. (1999). Opinions/perspectives/beliefs: Nature as professional resource–A new ecological approach to helping. *Kansas Chapter NASW News, 24*(2), 15.

Bodian, S. (1995). Simple in means, rich in ends: An interview with Arne Naess. In G. Sessions (Ed.), *Deep ecology for the 21st century: Readings on the philosophy and practice of the new environmentalism* (pp. 26-36). Boston: Shambhala.

Bookchin, M. (1986). *The modern crisis.* Philadelphia: New Society Publishers.

Canda, E. R. (1989). Religious content in social work education: A comparative approach. *Journal of Social Work Education, 25*(1), 36-45.

Canda, E. R. (1991). East/west philosophical synthesis in transpersonal theory. *Journal of Sociology and Social Welfare, 18*(4), 137-152.

Canda, E. R. (1996). Does religion and spirituality have a significant place in the core HBSE curriculum? Yes. In M. Bloom & W. Klein (Eds.), *Controversial issues in human behavior in the social environment* (pp. 172-177; 183-184). Boston: Allyn & Bacon.

Canda, E. R. (1997). Spirituality. *Encyclopedia of social work: 1997 supplement* (19th ed.). Washington, DC: National Association of Social Workers.

Canda, E. R., & Furman, L. D. (1999). *Spiritual diversity in social work practice: The heart of helping.* New York: The Free Press.

Capra, F. (1983). *The turning point: Science, society, and the rising culture.* New York: Bantam Books.

Carson, R. (1962). *Silent spring.* Boston: Houghton Mifflin.

Coates J. (1999). *The ecological crisis: Implications for social work.* Unpublished paper, St. Thomas University, Fredericton, NB, Canada.

Coates, J., & McKay, M. (1995). Toward a new pedagogy for social transformation. *Journal of Progressive Human Services, 6*(1), 27-44.

Cowley, A. S. (1993). Transpersonal social work: A theory for the 1990s. *Social Work, 38*(5), 527-534.

Cowley, A. S. (1996). Transpersonal social work. In F. J. Turner (Ed.), *Social work treatment: Interlocking theoretical approaches* (4th edition, pp. 663-698). New York: The Free Press.

Cowley, A. S., & Derezotes, D. (1994). Transpersonal psychology and social work education. *Journal of Social Work Education, 30*(1), 32-41.

DeJong, P., & Miller, S. D. (1995). How to interview for client strengths. *Social Work, 40*(6), 729-736.

Derezotes, D. S., & Evans, K. E. (1995). Spirituality and religiosity in practice: In-depth interviews of social work practitioners. *Social Thought, 18*(1), 39-56.

Devall, B., & Sessions, G. (1985). *Deep ecology.* Salt Lake City: Peregrine Smith Books.

diZerega, G. (1996). A critique of Ken Wilber's account of deep ecology and nature religions. *Trumpeter, 13*(2), 52-71.

Drengson, A. R. (1995). The deep ecology movement. *Trumpeter, 12*(3), 143-145.

Drengson, A. R., & Inoue, Y. (Eds.). (1995). *The deep ecology movement: An introductory anthology.* Berkeley: North Atlantic Press.

Fleck-Henderson, A. (1993). A constructivist approach to human behavior and the social environment. *Journal of Teaching in Social Work, 8*(1/2), 219-239.

Fox, W. (1984). Deep ecology: A new philosophy of our time? *The Ecologist, 14*(5/6), 194-200.

Fox, W. (1990). Transpersonal ecology: Psychologizing ecophilosophy. *The Journal of Transpersonal Psychology, 22*(1), 59-96.

Fox, W. (1995). *Toward a transpersonal ecology: Developing new foundations for environmentalism.* New York: State University of New York Press.

Granvold, D. K. (1996). Constructivist psychotherapy. *Families in Society, 77*(6), 345-359.

Gutierrez, L. M. (1994). Beyond coping: An empowerment perspective on stressful life events. *The Journal of Sociology and Social Welfare, 21*(3), 201-219.

Gutierrez, L. M., DeLois, K. A., & GlenMaye, L. (1995). The organizational context of empowerment practice: Implications for social work administration. *Social Work, 40*(2), 249-258.

Harman, W. (1998). *Global mind change: The promise of the 21st century* (2nd ed.). San Francisco: Berrett-Koehler Publishers.

Hoff, M. D., & McNutt, J. G. (Eds.). (1994). The global environmental crisis: Implications for social welfare and social work. Brookfield, VT: Ashgate Publishing.

Hoff, M. D., & Polack, R. (1993). Social dimensions of the environmental crisis: Challenges for social work. *Social Work, 38*(2), 204-211.

Hutchison, E. D. (1999). *Dimensions of human behavior: Person and environment.* Thousand Oaks, CA: Pine Forge Press.

Imre, R. W. (1982). *Knowing and caring: Philosophical issues in social work.* New York: University Press of America.

Kaluger, G., & Kaluger, M. F. (1984). *Human development: The span of life.* St. Louis: Times Mirror/Mosby.

LaChapelle, D. (1995). Ritual–the pattern that connects. In G. Sessions (Ed.), *Deep ecology for the 21st century: Readings on the philosophy and practice of the new environmentalism* (pp. 57-63). Boston: Shambhala.

Leopold, A. (1949). *A Sand County almanac: And sketches here and there.* New York: Oxford University Press.

List, P. C. (1993). *Radical environmentalism: Philosophy and tactics.* Belmont, CA: Wadsworth Publishing.

Macy, J. (1995). Working with environmental despair. In T. Roszak, M. Gomes, & A. Kanner (Eds.), *Ecopsychology: Restoring the earth-healing the mind* (pp. 240-259). San Francisco: Sierra Club Books.

Maslow, A. H. (1954). *Motivation and personality.* New York: Harper and Brothers.

Maslow, A. H. (1971). *The further reaches of human nature.* New York: The Viking Press.

McLaughlin, A. (1987). The critique of humanity and nature: Three recent philosophical reflections. *Trumpeter, 4*(4), 1-6.

McLaughlin, A. (1993). *Regarding nature: Industrialism and deep ecology.* Albany, NY: State University of New York Press.

McLaughlin, A. (1995). For a radical ecocentrism. In A. Drengson & Y. Inoue (Eds.), *The deep ecology movement: An introductory anthology* (pp. 257-280). Berkeley: North Atlantic Press.

Merchant, C. (1992). *Radical ecology: The search for a livable world.* New York: Routledge.

Murphy, M. (1998). On evolution and transformative practice: In appreciation of Ken Wilber. In D. Rothberg & S. Kelly (Eds.), *Ken Wilber in dialogue: Conversations with leading transpersonal thinkers* (pp. 53-61). Wheaton, IL: Quest Books.

Naess, A. (1973). The shallow and the deep, long range ecology movement. *Inquiry, 16*(2), 95-100.

Naess, A. (1984). A defense of the deep ecology movement. *Environmental Ethics, 6*(3), 265-270.

Naess, A. (1988). Identification as a source of deep ecological attitudes. In M. Tobias (Ed.), *Deep ecology* (pp. 256-270). San Marcos, CA: Avant Publishing.

Naess, A. (1989). *Ecology, community and lifestyle: Outline of an ecosophy.* New York: Cambridge University Press.

Naess, A. (1995a). The shallow and the deep, long-range ecology movement: A summary. In A. Drengson & Y. Inoue (Eds.), *The deep ecology movement: An introductory anthology* (pp. 3-9). Berkeley: North Atlantic Books.

Naess, A. (1995b). Deepness of questions and the deep ecology movement. In G. Sessions (Ed.), *Deep ecology for the 21st century: Readings on the philosophy and practice of the new environmentalism* (pp. 204-212). Boston: Shambhala.

Naess, A. (1995c). The deep ecological movement: Some philosophical aspects. In G Sessions (Ed.), *Deep ecology for the 21st century: Readings on the philosophy and practice of the new environmentalism* (pp. 64-84). Boston: Shambhala.

Naess, A. (1995d). The systematization of the logically ultimate norms and hypotheses of ecosophy T. In A. Drengson & Y. Inoue (Eds.), *The deep ecology movement: An introductory anthology* (pp. 31-48). Berkeley: North Atlantic Books.

Naess, A. (1995e). The deep ecology "eight points" revisited. In G. Sessions (Ed.), *Deep ecology for the 21st century: Readings on the philosophy and practice of the new environmentalism* (pp. 213-221). Boston: Shambhala.

Naess, A. (1995f). Politics and the ecological crisis: An introductory note. In G. Sessions (Ed.), *Deep ecology for the 21st century: Readings on the philosophy and practice of the new environmentalism* (pp. 445-453). Boston: Shambhala.

Okun, B. F. (1997). *Effective helping: Interviewing and counseling techniques* (5th ed.). New York: Brooks/Cole Publishing.

Park, K. M. (1996). The personal is ecological: Environmentalism of social work. *Social Work, 41*(3), 320-322.

Robbins, S. P., Chatterjee, P., & Canda, E. R. (1998). *Contemporary human behavior theory: A critical perspective for social work.* Boston: Allyn and Bacon.

Roberts, R. (1990). *Lessons from the past: Issues for social work theory.* New York: Tavistock Routledge.

Rothberg, D. (1998). Ken Wilber and the future of transpersonal inquiry: An introduction to the conversation. In D. Rothberg & S. Kelly (Eds.), *Ken Wilber in dialogue:*

Conversations with leading transpersonal thinkers (pp. 1-29). Wheaton, IL: Quest Books.

Rothberg, D., & Kelly, S. (Eds.). (1998). *Ken Wilber in dialogue: Conversations with leading transpersonal thinkers.* Wheaton, IL: Quest Books.

Rothenberg, D. (1993). *Is it painful to think?: Conversations with Arne Naess.* Minneapolis: University of Minnesota Press.

Russel, R. (1998). Spirituality and religion in graduate social work education. *Social Thought, 18*(2), 15-29.

Saleebey, D. (1991). Technological fix: Altering the consciousness of the social work profession. *Journal of Sociology and Social Welfare, 18*(4), 51-67.

Saleebey, D. (1996). The strengths perspective in social work practice: Extensions and cautions. *Social Work, 41*(3), 296-305.

Schriver, J. M. (1998). *Human behavior and the social environment: Shifting paradigms in essential knowledge for social work practice.* Boston: Allyn and Bacon.

Sessions, G. (1992). Arne Naess and the union of theory and practice. *Trumpeter, 9*(1), 73-76.

Sessions, G. (Ed.). (1995a). *Deep ecology for the 21st century: Readings on the philosophy and practice of the new environmentalism.* Boston: Shambhala.

Sessions, G. (1995b). Preface. In G. Sessions (Ed.), *Deep ecology for the 21st century: Readings on the philosophy and practice of the new environmentalism* (pp. ix-xxviii). Boston: Shambhala.

Smith, E., & Gray, C. (1995). Integrating and transcending divorce: A transpersonal model. *Social Thought, 18*(1), 57-74.

Turner, J. (1995). In wildness is the preservation of the world. In G. Sessions (Ed.), *Deep ecology for the 21st century: Readings on the philosophy and practice of the new environmentalism.* Boston: Shambhala.

Van Den Berg, N. (Ed.). (1995). *Feminist practice in the 21st century.* Washington: NASW Press.

Vaughn, F. (1980). Transpersonal psychotherapy: Context, content and process. In R. Walsh & F. Vaughn (Eds.), *Beyond ego: Transpersonal dimensions in psychology* (pp. 160-165). Los Angeles: Tarcher/Perigree.

Vaughn, F. (1995). *Shadows of the sacred: Seeing through spiritual illusions.* Wheaton, IL: Quest Books.

Walsh, R. N. (1984). Transpersonal psychology. In N. Sunberg & C. Keutzer (Eds.), *The encyclopedia of psychology* (pp. 459-481). Baltimore: Williams and Wilkins.

Walsh, R. N. (1998). Developmental and evolutionary synthesis in the recent writings of Ken Wilber. In D. Rothberg & S. Kelly (Eds.), *Ken Wilber in dialogue: Conversations with leading transpersonal thinkers* (pp. 30-52). Wheaton, IL: Quest Books.

Walsh, R. N., & Vaughan, F. (1980). *Beyond ego: Transpersonal dimensions in psychology.* Los Angeles: J. P. Tarcher.

Warren, K., Franklin, C., & Streeter, C. L. (1998). New directions in systems theory: Chaos and complexity. *Social Work, 43*(4), 357-372.

Weick, A. (1981). Reframing the person-in-environment perspective. *Social Work, 26*(2), 140-143.

Weick, A. (1987). Reconceptualizing the philosophical perspective of social work. *Social Service Review, 61*(2), 218-230.

Weick, A. (1991). The place of science in social work. *The Journal of Sociology and Social Welfare, 18*(4), 13-34.

Wilber, K. (1977). *The spectrum of consciousness.* Wheaton, IL: The Theosophical Publishing House.

Wilber, K. (1981). *Up from Eden.* New York: Doubleday/Anchor.

Wilber, K. (1983). *Eye to eye: The quest for the new paradigm.* Garden City, NY: Anchor Books.

Wilber, K. (1986). *A sociable God.* Boston: Shambhala.

Wilber, K. (1993). *Grace and grit: Spirituality and healing in the life and death of Treya Killiam Wilber.* Boston: Shambhala.

Wilber, K. (1995). *Sex, ecology, spirituality: The spirit of evolution.* Boston: Shambhala.

Wilber, K. (1996). *A brief history of everything.* Boston: Shambhala

Wilber, K. (1998). *The essential Ken Wilber: An introductory reader.* Boston: Shambhala.

Zimmerman, M. E. (1990). Deep ecology and ecofeminism: The emerging dialogue. In I. Diamond & G. Orenstein (Eds.), *Reweaving the world: The emergence of ecofeminism* (pp. 138-154). San Francisco: Sierra Club Books.

Zimmerman, M. E. (1994). *Contesting earth's future: Radical ecology and postmodernity.* Berkeley: University of California Press.

Zimmerman, M. E. (1998). A transpersonal diagnosis of the ecological crisis. In D. Rothberg & S. Kelly (Eds.), *Ken Wilber in dialogue: Conversations with leading transpersonal thinkers* (pp. 180-206). Wheaton, IL: Quest Books.

Alleviating Suffering in the Face of Death: Insights from Constructivism and a Transpersonal Narrative Approach

Elizabeth D. Smith

SUMMARY. Confronting one's mortality is at the heart of much human suffering. Building upon her previous development and testing of an exploratory model of psychospiritual distress, the author explores the confrontation of death in light of a transpersonal narrative with four new dimensions: (a) normalization of death, (b) divine intention, i.e., a belief in a supernatural force of higher power that provides a cosmic order, (c) surrender, i.e., the ability to let go of the outcome of events and to accept the unknown, and (d) transpersonal existence, i.e., a belief in a continued existence beyond the known mortal self. Through a constructivist perspective on this transpersonal narrative, one can understand how personal reality is constructed and how affect flows from core beliefs that mediate events. This offers an explanatory model of how annihilation vulnerability of personhood can be mediated, resulting in diminished

Elizabeth D. Smith, DSW, is Associate Professor at the National Catholic School of Social Service, The Catholic University of America. Research support for the development of the conceptual model of suffering in the face of death was provided through a grant at the Johns Hopkins Oncology Center by the Nathan Cummings Foundation, Inc. (E-mail: smithe@cua.edu).

Gratitude is extended to my colleague, Dr. Barbara Peo Early, for her numerous hours of vigorous clarifying debate of the concepts, and her expert critique of the appropriate usage of cognitive and constructivist theory.

[Haworth co-indexing entry note]: "Alleviating Suffering in the Face of Death: Insights from Constructivism and a Transpersonal Narrative Approach." Smith, Elizabeth D. Co-published simultaneously in *Social Thought* (The Haworth Press, Inc.) Vol. 20, No. 1/2, 2001, pp. 45-61; and: *Transpersonal Perspectives on Spirituality in Social Work* (ed: Edward R. Canda, and Elizabeth D. Smith) The Haworth Press, Inc. 2001, pp. 45-61. Single or multiple copies of this article are available for a fee from The Haworth Document Delivery Service [1-800-342-9678, 9:00 a.m. - 5:00 p.m. (EST). E-mail address: getinfo@haworthpressinc.com].

45

suffering. It suggests implications for practice to alleviate the actual suffering a person experiences. *[Article copies available for a fee from The Haworth Document Delivery Service: 1-800-342-9678. E-mail address: <getinfo@haworthpressinc.com> Website: <http://www.Haworth Press.com> © 2001 by The Haworth Press, Inc. All rights reserved.]*

KEYWORDS. Transpersonal, death, anxiety, spirituality, social work

INTRODUCTION

Addressing psychospiritual distress associated with the threat of death is an important, and yet neglected, issue for social work practice. Confronting one's mortality is at the heart of much human suffering. In an effort to understand suffering among cancer patients, this author developed and tested an explanatory model of psychospiritual distress from a transpersonal perspective which revealed that those patients who had a higher level of transpersonal development, especially a normalized view of death, were less distressed (Smith, 1993; Smith, 1995). Factor analysis of new data helped to identify four dimensions of a distress-relieving transpersonal perspective as: (a) normalization of death, conceptually defined as the ability to tolerate the comprehension of personal mortality and to view death as part of the normal life cycle, (b) divine intention, conceptually defined as a belief in a supernatural force or higher power that provides a cosmic order, (c) surrender, or the ability to let go of the outcome of events and to accept the unknown, (d) transpersonal existence, conceptualized as a belief in a continued existence beyond the known mortal self; for some this would be a belief in a spirit-self or soul.

These empirical observations led the author to reformulate an understanding of suffering and response to death within a perspective that blends insights from constructivism and transpersonal theory. From a constructivist paradigm, the possibility of suffering is inherent in the threat of death, yet suffering is not inevitable. Suffering is not the equivalent of fear. While fear is an affect, suffering is an interpretive cognition. Fear in the face of death is instinctive and inevitable, biologically linked to self-preservation. Suffering is the interpretation of a threat to a person's integrity, their "I am-ness." Suffering persists so long as the threat of annihilation of personhood persists or until the response is transformed by alternative spiritual interpretive meaning. Therefore, interpretation may or may not lead to suffering. It is the very interpretative nature and spiritual context of suffering that sets it apart from physical pain and psychological distress. The purpose of this article is to theoretically explicate this re-formulated understanding of suffering within a constructivist paradigm.

CONSTRUCTIVIST AND TRANSPERSONAL INSIGHTS ON SUFFERING

The constructivist paradigm maintains that "knowledge is a human con-struction, never certifiable as ultimately true but problematic and ever chang-ing" (Guba, 1990, p. 26). Within this paradigm, one must take a position of relativism, of an openness to the continuing search for ever more sophisticated constructions. Constructivism is how people make meaning of their lives through their perceptions, the cognitive and affective operations of the mind (Berger & Luckman, 1966; Franklin, 1995). These constructed meanings give way to multiple realities, realities that exist in people's minds. Thus individu-als actively create and construe their personal and social realities (Brower, 1996; Granvold, 1996; Guba, 1990).

Constructivism epistemologically adopts a motor theory of the mind in which the mind is a dynamic constructive machine capable of not only produc-ing its own output, but also in large part, producing its input as well. Thus, knowledge is an evolutionary result of an interactive process between the ex-ternal event and the interpretations imposed upon the event (Granvold, 1996). Because the constructivist paradigm takes the ontological position of relativ-ism, in which human reality exists in the form of multiple mental construc-tions, it must necessarily take the epistemological position of subjectivism as the means of unlocking the constructions held by individuals (Guba,1990).

Therefore, in methods for inquiring into these reality constructions, individ-ual constructions must be elicited and refined hermeneutically in a dialectical process with "the aim of producing as informed and sophisticated a construc-tion as possible" (Guba, 1990, p. 26). In contrast to realism, where there is an assumption of a valid, objective, and knowable reality, constructivism relies on viability rather than validity. The viability of a conceptualized personal re-ality is determined by the function it serves for the individual who adopts it, as he or she fits within an overall personal and social system of belief into which the personal belief is incorporated (Granvold, 1996). Such viability becomes all important to the alleviation of suffering. It is just such a viable system of thought that mediates between perceived life-threatening events and the level of suffering experienced by the person. When the viability of the construction is shaken, the individual suffers, and continues to suffer until such time when a newly viable construction is formulated.

Death and Human Suffering as Narrative

According to Cassell (1982), personhood is key to understanding the source of suffering. However, one usually defines oneself, by role in relationship to other, such as daughter, friend, coworker, or spouse. These role definitions are central to one's identity or personhood. Whenever the intactness of that identity or the integrity of personhood is threatened, there is suffering (Byock, 1994; 1996). The threat to integrity of personhood, however, is one of interpretation and individual mental constructions of identity and wholeness:

> The death of the self has many possible meanings. It can be viewed as an ending, as a beginning, as a transition or rite of passage, or as all three. It can be viewed as a reward or as a punishment or as partaking of both. It can be perceived as a base from which a series of losses develop: loss of people, loss of experiencing, loss of control, loss of competence, loss of capacity to complete plans and projects, loss of body, loss of things. (Kalish, 1980, p. 82)

The anticipation of death is experienced within a complex web of cultural and religious meanings (Koenig & Gates-Williams, 1995). The meanings by which individuals contextualize themselves or form their sense of personhood may be described as their personal narrative. Narrative is the basic way that individuals organize their life experiences over time in a meaningful way. "Narratives provide structures of meaning that allow the person to understand both the role and the wider social or cultural plot of which it is a part" (Niemeyer & Stewart, 1996, p. 361). Problems occur when narratives no longer reflect an individual's lived experience or are no longer viable, so that a person gets lost because he or she has no "road map" to follow. The individual's narrative begins to disintegrate because he or she is unable to "emplot" and integrate new phenomena. This threat to the narrative wholeness of the self-concept results in anxiety as the person is unable to make sense of some event in the world (Niemeyer & Stewart, 1996, p. 361).

Death is an ego-transcending phenomenon for which humans may not have a viable narrative framework. For many, it is a universal event that seems senseless, because accepting the reality of death is not taught in American culture. According to Foos-Graber (1989), "the death moment has been forgotten by our society. Rather than accepting death as the culmination of life, we see it as a tragic inevitability" (p. 3). In fact, foreign medical visitors have often commented on "the apparent belief of many Americans that death is just one more disease to be conquered, a tenacious but not invincible foe" (Callahan, 1995). Western medicine has become engaged in a relentless pursuit of death prevention through ever-advancing technology. In this context, death is viewed as a failure of medicine. Psychospiritually, however, the ultimate supremacy of death is problematic:

> The human problem: Having a mind, being a body, is nowhere quite so painfully and clearly apparent as in medicine. Painful, because to be a body means you must die. Clear because to have a mind means that you know this. (Keizer, 1994, p. 1)

Caught up in the materialism espoused by the medical model, Westerners have failed to understand what many Easterners accept: to prevent death one would have to prevent birth. When Shakyamuni Buddha was asked, "What is the cause of aging and death?," he answered, "Birth is the cause of aging and death." Death defines life, and it is unique to the human condition to have an awareness of this:

> The truth is that the consciousness of death is a peculiar privilege of humankind. Other mortal beings, it would seem, have only the briefest awareness of death as an approaching reality, if indeed they have this. Apprehension of death, therefore, is one of the qualities distinguishing humans from the lower animals; it is to be considered a mark of higher intelligence. Still, because of this blessing, we often become obsessed with the fear of death and even go to absurd extremes to avoid it. (Daisaku Ikeda, 1995, p. 16)

Most people cannot tolerate the notion of their own death. It has been said that looking at your own death is like trying to look at the sun; you can only do it for a few seconds at a time and then you have to look away. Freud questioned the ability of the ego to contemplate its own non-existence and noted that "our unconscious does not believe in its own death; it behaves as if immortal" (Freud, 1915 in Freud, 1959, p. 304). Because death is counter to ego-existence, it is perceived as a threat to the integrity of the person and the result is suffering:

> Your ego is a set of thoughts that define your universe. It's like a familiar room built of thoughts; you see the universe through its windows. You are secure in it, but to the extent that you are afraid to venture outside, it has become a prison. Your ego has you conned. You believe you need its specific thoughts to survive. The ego controls you through your fear of loss of identity. To give up these thoughts, it seems, would eliminate you, and so you cling to them. (Ram Dass, 1980, p. 139)

These constructions to which one clings, including apprehension of death, are most often negatively framed as an enemy to the ego. A personal narrative within which to frame the reality of death is actually difficult to construct, as death is not typically associated with any preexisting sense of self, nor any psychological roles or situated identities that individuals have enacted in previous life contexts. Thus, death does not allow for the individual's awareness of his or her identity, continuity, and self-images formed through role enactment, and emplotted into comprehensible narrative based on experience (Neimeyer & Stewart, 1996). Rather, one might ask:

> ... are not the thoughts of dying often turned towards the practical painful, obscure, visceral aspect, towards the "seamy side" of death which is, as it happens, the side that death actually presents to them and forces them to feel and which far more closely resembles a crushing burden, a difficulty in breathing, a destroying thirst, than the abstract idea to which we are accustomed to give the Death? (Spiegel & Tristman, 1997, p. 131)

The "crushing burden" one experiences is the negative narrative constructed out of fear of annihilation of personhood. Death of the ego is incomprehensible. Suffering of the ego is inevitable.

The Transpersonal Narrative

Concepts from transpersonal theory challenge the commonly held assumptions that: "(a) linear rational thinking is the standard for optimal cognitive development; (b) autonomy is the standard for psychosocial maturity; and (c) ordinary waking consciousness is the standard for normal mental operation" (Canda, 1994, p. 138). Rather, transpersonal psychology posits four basic tenets: (a) consciousness, (b) conditioning, (c) personality, and (d) identity (Walsh & Vaughan, 1982). These tenets are essential to understanding a transpersonal view of personhood.

Consciousness is usually viewed as a "defensively contracted state," whereas optimum consciousness is viewed as being greater and potentially available at any time. Any one state of consciousness is thereby limited, and to awaken to any one single reality is to recognize its relativity. Conditioning, from the transpersonal perspective, is the entrapment of people within their own conditioning. However, they may escape from this entrapment. One form of conditioning is attachment, which is central to suffering, and letting go of this attachment is the means to cease one's suffering. Personality is not given a central role, but rather it is given relatively less importance. Instead of trying to modify the personality, the goal is to shift away from an exclusive identification with it. And finally, identity in the transpersonal orientation is viewed as the process by which something is experienced as self. Identification with internal processes tends to be more significant than identification with the external. It is maintained that an individual is dominated by everything with which he or she identifies (Smith, 1995). A transpersonal narrative, then, would serve to alleviate suffering by incorporating an optimum view of consciousness, an escape from the entrapment of conditioning, a shifting away from an exclusive identity with the personality, and a disidentification from all with which one has been previously identified.

This transpersonal narrative would create a cognitive structure to enable a tolerance of an acute awareness of the vulnerability of personhood to annihilation through assignment of spiritual meaning to that awareness. This narrative encourages meaningful interpersonal attachments, and yet allows the cognitive ability to disattach and experience the dissolution of the boundaries of the self.

Cognitive structure. Cognitive theory (Beck, 1976) flows from the constructivist world view and assumes the mediational position in which "cognitive activity mediates the responses the individual has to his or her environment, and to some extent dictates the degree of adjustment or maladjustment of the individual" (Dobson & Block, 1988, p. 29). Thus, a stimulus is screened and interpreted through the lens of thinking patterns. Events in one's life are understood within this mediating context that constitutes a personal narrative (Neimeyer & Stewart, 1996; Sarbin, 1986). When a person experiences a traumatic event (the confrontation of one's personal mortality) and through the meaning-making process develops a negative role, "a new narrative (trauma narrative) and self (traumatized self) emerge" (Neimeyer & Stewart, 1996, p. 362). When one does not have an adequate narrative in which to make sense or meaning of a life event, anxiety results (Kelly, 1955). Death confrontation may represent such an event in which a person's personal or spiritual narrative is inadequate to contextualize the event, resulting in psychospiritual distress.

Annihilation vulnerability of personhood. According to object relations theory, humans have, at core, three primitive fears (Cassidy, 1999; Goldstein, 1995). The third most primitive fear is of the loss of the love of the object; with this fear, one believes that his or her primary love object will cease to love him or her. From an infant's point of view, this would be fear of the loss of the love of the mother or mothering object. The second most primitive fear is loss of the object. In this case, one believes that the loved one will be lost, and, therefore, they are afraid. From an infant's point of view, this would be fear of the loss of the mother or mothering object. The first most primitive fear is fear of annihilation. Fear of annihilation is the belief that one will be annihilated or cease to exist. Infants are entirely dependent on the caretaking of a mothering object. Without this caretaking, the infant would literally be annihilated or cease to be. If the mother or mothering object is lost, the infant will have no caretaker and thus would be annihilated. If the mother ceases to love the infant and does not perform the caretaking role, the infant will eventually be annihilated. While fear of loss of the object and fear of loss of the love of the object are epigenetically more distinct, they are ultimately no more than increasingly subtle versions of fear of annihilation. Each individual, having been an infant, has these three primitive cognitive structures, in all their permutations, which underlie all fear. Essentially, each person is vulnerable to annihilation anxiety so long as one believes that personhood is subject to possible destruction through physical death.

Spiritual meaning. Spiritual meaning within the narrative results in a quieting of the mind. This ability can be cultivated throughout a lifetime and can be constructed contextually by the individual's personal belief system. These personal constructs are usually formed through early socialization into a collectively held cultural or religious belief. The practice of resting in great equanimity or achieving a steady inner peace is key, no matter what context that practice takes. The cultural or religious methods of practice that lead to spiritual meaning are ultimately of little consequence so long as one is able to obtain it. Spiritual meaning also contributes to individuals' transcending suffering in the face of death because they no longer believe in a fearful outcome.

> People who are not afraid of dying are people who have tamed their mind, those who have actually practiced letting their mind rest quietly, in great equanimity. Then, when they die, they can do that and it gives them a chance to rise above their karmic predisposition and not be blown about helplessly. This is true for people who have done great meditation in any of the religions of the world, be it Catholicism, Judaism, Islam, Buddhism, or whatever. (Giorno, 1996)

Spiritual meaning disempowers the threat inherent in the annihilation vulnerability of personhood. As Ram Dass (1996) recounts:

> Once the inner connection to that which does not die is strong enough, it can withstand great opposing forces. There is an old story about a conquering army going through villages, and killing and pillaging as it went. The soldiers caused terror in the hearts of the people in the countryside. The army was especially harsh with the monks they found in the monasteries, not only humiliating them, but often disemboweling them. There was one particularly harsh army captain, who was infamous for his cruelty. He arrived in one town and asked his adjutant for a report, about the people in the town. The adjutant reported: "All the people are very frightened of you and are bowing down to you." This gave the captain pleasure. Then the adjutant continued, "In the local monastery all the monks have fled to the mountains in terror . . . except for one monk." Hearing that, the captain became furious about this one monk and rushed to the

monastery. He pushed open the gates, and there in the middle of the courtyard was the monk, just standing there. The captain walked up to him and he said in his most haughty manner, "Don't you know who I am? Why I could take my sword and run it through your belly without blinking an eye!" "And don't you know who I am?" replied the monk, gently. "I could have your sword run through my belly without blinking an eye." It is said that the captain, recognizing the greater truth of the moment, sheathed his sword, bowed, and left. (p. 11)

Dissolution of the boundaries of the self. Spiritual traditions have many forms of dissolving or transcending the self and moving beyond a sense of a separate self, such as transcendent surrender through devotional practices, prayer, profound rituals, or vision quests. A repeated inquiry into the question of "Who am I?" is one such practice to achieving the dissolution of the self (Kornfield, 1993).

A Lutheran minister speaking at a thanatology conference a number of years ago told the participants in his workshop the ten most important questions he asked the AIDS patients he was working with in New York City. He suggested the participants write them down. "The first question," he said, "is 'Who am I?' " After a silent pause, he went on. "The second question is, 'Who am I?' " He paused again, "The third question is, 'Who am I?' " After the third time, the workshop participants giggled and commented to each other, realizing the repetition of the question. But the minister did not smile. He continued, deliberately asking the question ten times. Each participant discovered after answering the question the first few times with role descriptions of self, such as mother, student, engineer, brother, dancer, etc., that he or she eventually ran out of roles and was left with a core self in relation only to self. With the "me," as defined by relationship, nearly completely dissolved, an individual is left with the revelation of the essence of self, the "I." The minister explained that this is what a person who is dying experiences–the dissolution of the social and psychological self. It was an instructive lesson in the stripping away of identity and aptly illustrates what the repeated inquiry has to teach.

Beyond the dissolution of the social and psychological self is "being cognition." Being cognition is a state, similar to cosmic consciousness, that is unifying, complete, and self-sufficient. It resolves dichotomies, polarities, and conflicts (Maslow, 1985). It is a state of complete disidentification:

> Since there is no longer any exclusive identification with anything, the me/not me dichotomy is transcended and such persons experience themselves as being both nothing and everything. They are both pure awareness (nothing) and the entire universe (everything). Being identified with both no location and all locations, nowhere and everywhere, they experi-

ence having transcended space and positionality. (Walsh & Vaughan, 1982, p. 52)

In this state, there is unity and cosmic wholeness.

MEDIATION OF DEATH CONFRONTATION
THROUGH THE TRANSPERSONAL NARRATIVE

Lack of a personal narrative that effectively mediates the realization of the annihilation vulnerability of personhood may well be the source of all suffering. This inability to cognitively construct a meaningful interpretation of painful events, either externally or internally induced, will deliver the individual into a dark realm *of psychospiritual distress.* This realm has been described by Washburn (1988) as "regression in the service of transcendence." Implicit in this description of suffering is the inherent possibility of growth, but not its inevitability. Attention to the finitude of self, whether forced upon an individual through either literal or perceived life-threatening circumstances, or intentionally sought through spiritual practice, brings the individual to a sense of the dissolution of the life and the initial darkness of utter annihilation. The metaphor of the night, taken from the writing of St. John of the Cross (Peers, 1977), described as a long period of unknowing, loss, and despair that must be traversed as a matter of self-emptying. This process can be terrifying.

> Now the dark night deepens. As our outer and inner worlds dissolve, we lose our sense of reference. There arises a great sense of unease and fear, leading students into a realm of fear and terror. "Where is there any security?" "Wherever I look, things are dissolving." In these stages we can experience the dissolution and dying within our own body. We may look down and see pieces of our body seeming to melt away and decay, as if we were a corpse. We can see ourselves dying, or having died, in a thousand ways, through illness, battles, and misfortune. At this point, other powerful visions can arise, visions of the death of others, visions of wars, dying armies, funeral pyres, or charnel grounds. . . . From this realm of terror and death arises a very deep realization of the suffering inherent in life: the suffering of pain, the suffering of the loss of pleasant things and, hanging over it all, the enormous suffering of the death of whatever is created or loved by us. (Kornfield, 1993, p. 149)

A constructivist explanation of the suffering response to death is found in the idea that cognitions are seen as both the cause and the effect of an experience, "that is, cognitions are influenced by past and present environmental input and also shape the environment by giving meaning and selecting actions to change it" (Berlin, 1982, p. 218). When individuals negatively interpret the meaning of events, they are often unable to cope. Information given by one's environment may be viewed as ambiguous, punitive, or overwhelming, as dependent upon Western societal views of death. Thus, circumstances of a situation along with personal factors such as beliefs and associated emotions determine an individual's response (Berlin, 1982). Thoughts of one's own death may cause suffering, but they may also be a result of suffering. From a cognitive constructivist's view, change in suffering ultimately occurs through alteration of thought patterns in the shaping of one's personal reality.

Commonly held thought patterns that seem to be associated with the least amount of suffering are found in four components of transpersonal narrative about death: normalization of death, divine intention, surrender, and transpersonal existence. These components were refined conceptually from earlier research (Smith, 1993; Smith, 1995). In the earlier studies, transpersonal development was found to be negatively correlated with psychosocial distress among cancer patients, indicating that higher levels of transpersonal narrative were related to lower suffering in the face of life-threatening illness (Smith, 1993). In considering what mediates the annihilation vulnerability resulting in the actual suffering an individual experiences, it may be helpful to examine these dimensions of transpersonal narratives about death.

Normalization of Death

As a component of transpersonal narrative, the ability to normalize one's own death is central. Individuals with a strong transpersonal narrative view death as a normal part of the life cycle, as one eternal round, as part of the life-death-rebirth loop, whether literally or figuratively. These individuals have constructed a narrative that has a natural place for death and hold a perspective of death that is comforting rather than distressing. They may envision themselves as sitting on the right hand of Jesus, as a memory to their children, as a vibrating ball of light, or as compost returning life to the earth. Constructively, they have been able to employ and integrate the phenomenon of death into a cultural narrative that satisfactorily converts this unexperienced event/state into a contextual understanding that, for them, makes the unknown known. The content of the narratives held by individuals will be as diverse as the individuals themselves, but the function of the narrative will be the same. Normalization of death functions as a means for the ego to transcend the possibility of its own total annihilation.

Divine Intention

Another component of a strong transpersonal narrative is that of divine intention. In this view, the universe or cosmos has a divine purpose, and it is ordered or structured by divine good. Whether or not that divinity takes the form of an anthropomorphized God, a supernatural force, a type of transcendent physics, an evolutionary model of spiritual development, or a great equanimity, something transcendent gives benevolent meaning to existence for these individuals. From this perspective, suffering has meaning and serves an ultimate purpose. Nothing is entirely senseless. Narratives of life adopted by individuals with a strong transpersonal narrative are contextualized with cultural variations of divine intention, giving inherent structures of meaning to the end of their lives. Individuals understand differently according to the way they define life and what philosophy or religious belief they adhere to. However, individuals maintaining a cognitive construction of divine intention do not accept a materialistic view of the universe devoid of transcendent realities. Instead, they exist within a constructed reality that allows for transcendental phenomena that order the world for cosmic purposes.

Surrender

Transpersonal means "beyond the person." Those with a strong transpersonal narrative know on some level that there is more to who they are than the ego-identified self, if they can but surrender the ego. Attachment is the perpetual obstacle to moments of surrender that contribute to individual suffering. In an effort to shift away from an exclusive identity with the personality and to surrender, individuals with a transpersonal narrative will attempt to transcend their attachments, sometimes through spiritual practice. One example is Buddhist mindfulness meditation:

> In mindfulness practice, self is experienced as a flow, a process, a rushing and teeming patterning that changes over time. A quiet mind free of thoughts, continual surrender into the moment, and relaxation of the constraints of false self all give the illusion of release from neurotic attachment. Yet these experiences, too, can become the basis for pride and attachment. The three objects of craving that the Buddha spoke about in his Second Noble Truth–sense pleasures, existence, and nonexistence–all are re-created in crystalline form in the progress of meditation so that the grasping after them can be identified. It is this grasping that the Buddha identified as the eradicable source of suffering, and meditation is designed to make this grasping familiar in all of its forms. (Epstein, 1995, p. 151)

In other forms of transpersonal narrative some individuals pray to God for deliverance, some try to exercise the will, some use insight meditation, some practice various forms of abstinence, some perform rituals, and so on. Whatever the manifestation of the practice, the goal is to transcend the appetite-based self and surrender the ego. It is a letting go of an attachment to the outcome of events, and an acceptance of the unknown. In this context, surrender is not reactive submission, but proactive acceptance. It serves an empowering function.

Transpersonal Existence

One of the strongest cognitive antidotes to annihilation vulnerability of personhood is the belief in existence beyond the mortal person. Positive constructs of the death state are the most helpful in mediating annihilation vulnerability and minimizing personal suffering. However, even negative constructs serve the ego in its attempt to survive regardless of the form that survival takes.

Kastenbaum (1975) describes the various ways in which the death state has been characterized by individual thinkers and different cultural traditions. First, there is *more of the same.* Death is a state that can have its crises and problems just as life before the death event. The deceased simply passes from one realm to another; however, this continuation is not identical with immortality. In this view, held by many tribal societies, death can happen again, as the dead can be destroyed. Second, death can be viewed as *perpetual development.* Many thinkers have been influenced by the theory of evolution to posit a universe in which the primary principle is development. The death state varies from person to person according to the progress to human fulfillment they have already made. Development will continue towards "awareness," "enlightenment," or "higher consciousness." The opportunity for perpetual development is available to all, but there are no guarantees. An individual can fail to develop both before and after death. Third, there is the notion of the death state as *less of the same.* This is a very common view of death in which the dead are "plunged into a dark pit from which there is no escape, only a gradual submergence. This is the 'underworld' of miserable shades whose . . . individual characteristics erode with time until all differentiation has disappeared" (p. 29). It is a "place where the dead subsist without joy or hope, mere wretched shadows and remnants of what they once had been" (p. 29). Fourth, death is conceived as a state of *waiting.* The dead are believed to be in some state of restful waiting. Waiting for the judgment day or the final disposition of the soul. They are "taking a good long rest" until they take their place for eternity. Fifth, one of the most traditional and popular views, but more radical for Westerners, is that of death as *recycling.* In this view, the core of one's being cannot be destroyed, but is perpetually reborn into multiple lives. It is the great wheel of life in which the individual experiences birth, death, and rebirth much like the rhythm of the seasons.

These are some of the ways in which individuals have constructed their reality around the death state. Individuals who hold the view of some form of transpersonal existence are better able to tolerate annihilation threats to personhood. By assuming that death is a state, we eliminate the idea of death as a non-state:

> It is very difficult to unthink and unspeak death as a state. Our needs for logical development and sheer cognitive affective comfort will find little nourishment in the barren, alien vision of a nonstate. We know little about nothing, and much prefer to convert nothing into anything. (Kastenbaum, 1975, p. 33)

Death as a state of "anything" engenders less ego-distress or suffering than the idea of death as "no-thing," not even a state. For in a non-state, the ego ceases to be.

IMPLICATIONS FOR PRACTICE

Social work practitioners are designated healers. They are engaged in the struggle against all suffering that manifests itself in the human condition. The professional goal is to alleviate suffering. Focusing on stressors in both the person and the environment, practice efforts may be directed at either large systemic ills in society or the maladaptive coping of individual clients. Wherever these efforts are directed, they must take into account the human construction of personal reality. What may be sources of suffering for some, may not prove to be suffering for others. It is important then to enter the individual's perception of reality and see his or her world from the inside out. Because there is some empirical evidence (Smith, 1993) revealing a relationship between strong transpersonal narrative and decreased suffering, it seems that exploring transpersonal narrative for avenues of strengthening that belief would be one means of alleviating suffering.

As a first step, a practitioner should assess the level of *annihilation vulnerability* the client is experiencing. Is it acute? Is it more subtle or disguised? Is the client experiencing direct fear of death or is there an underlying existential anxiety? How safe does the client perceive himself or herself to be? Has there been a triggering event, a life-threatening diagnosis, a near accident, a traumatic experience, or a realization of finitude brought on by a life transition such as divorce or retirement? What is the symptomatology expressing the annihilation vulnerability? Are the mediating constructions held by the client helpful in managing the acute awareness of the annihilation vulnerability of personhood that has been triggered?

Secondly, it is important to explore the component constructions of transpersonal narrative as outlined above. What are the client's beliefs about death? What cultural context was he or she given regarding death? Is his or her personal death perspective one that is comforting rather than distressing? How well does the client's learned belief system regarding death hold up in the face of death's perceived actuality? Does the client find order in the universe? Does he or she believe in God or a supernatural force? What gives life, and thereby death, its meaning? Wherein does he or she find purpose for being? Are there lessons to be learned in suffering? Can surrender be helpful? What does surrender imply to the client? What attachments cause the client suffering? How does the client move beyond the self in times of suffering? What are the client's beliefs regarding death as a state? Does the client conceive of an existence beyond this existence and, if so, does that serve as a source of comfort to the client?

Next, it is useful to work cooperatively with the client in constructing or reconstructing viable components of transpersonal narrative that mediate suffering in the current situation. Although the stressors that may lead to suffering cannot always be eliminated, the perception of the impact of those stressors as sources of suffering can be affected by cognitive and spiritual restructuring. Social workers never cease to fight the causes of suffering or necessarily accept the inevitability of death. However, when all efforts are being made on every front to fight the causes, practitioners can also work with a client's individually constructed realities to create a source of solace for that individual. Social work should not be content to work with individuals to accept conditions that lead to suffering, putting the responsibility on the individual to bear the burden. But whatever burdens the individual is forced to continue to bear, let the practitioner be a supportive guide within that individual's inner world in co-constructing a comforting reality.

Finally, it would be vital to connect the client to ongoing supportive resources that will foster continued transpersonal development. However the client defines those sources for himself or herself, linking the client to these resources will serve as a mediating structure to alleviate psychospiritual distress associated with further annihilation threats to personhood.

CONCLUSION

The confrontation of death has been explored in light of a transpersonal narrative with four dimensions: (a) normalization of death, i.e., the ability to tolerate the comprehension of personal mortality and to view death as part of the normal life cycle; (b) divine intention, i.e., a belief in a supernatural force of higher power that provides a cosmic order; (c) surrender, i.e., the ability to let go of the outcome of events and to accept the unknown; and; (d) transpersonal existence, i.e., a belief in a continued existence beyond the known mortal self–for some this would be a belief in a spirit-self or soul. By employing a constructivist perspective on this transpersonal narrative, one can understand how personal reality is constructed and how affect flows from core beliefs that mediate events. The components of transpersonal narrative about death suggested here offer an explanatory model of how annihilation vulnerability of personhood can be mediated, resulting in diminished suffering. This explanatory model suggests implications for practice that may lead to interventions to alleviate the actual suffering a person experiences.

REFERENCES

Beck, A. (1976). *Cognitive-Therapy and Emotional Disorders.* New York: Penguin Books.

Berger, P., & Luckman, T. (1966). *The Social Construction of Reality.* Garden City, NY: Doubleday.

Berlin, S. (1982). Cognitive behavioral interventions for social work practice. *Social Work, 27*(3), 218-26.

Brower, A. (1996). Group development as constructed social reality revisited: The constructivism of small groups. *Families in Society: The Journal of Contemporary Human Services, 77*(6), 336-344.

Byock, I. (1994). When suffering persists. *Journal of Palliative Care, 102,* 8-31.

Byock, I. (1996). *The nature of suffering and the nature of opportunity at the end of life.* Unpublished paper.

Callahan, D. (1995). Frustrated mastery: The cultural context of death in America. In *Caring for Patients at the End of Life* [Special Issue]. *Western Journal of Medicine, 163,* 226-230.

Canda, E. (1994). East/west philosophical synthesis in transpersonal theory. *Journal of Sociology and Social Welfare, 18*(4), 137-152.

Cassell, E. (1982). The nature of suffering and the goals of medicine. *New England Journal of Medicine, 306*(11), 639-645.

Daisaku Ikeda. (1995). The nature of death. *Seiko Times, 406,* 16-29.

Dass, R. (1996, June). *Work with the dying.* Unpublished paper taken from his forthcoming book on consciousness and aging. Presented at The Caregiver's Inner Life Conference at the Fetzer Institute, Kalamazoo, MI.

Dass, R. (1980). Relative realities. In R. Walsh & F. Vaughan, (Eds.), *Beyond ego; Transpersonal dimensions in psychotherapy* (pp. 138-141). New York: Jeremy Tarcher, Inc.

Dobson, K., & Block, L. (1988). Historical and philosophical bases of the cognitive-behavioral therapies. In K. Dobson (Ed), *Handbook of Cognitive-Behavioral Therapies* (pp. 3-338). New York: Guilford.

Epstein, M. (1995). *Thoughts without a thinker.* New York: Basic Books.

Franklin, C. (1995). Expanding the vision of the social constructionist debates: creating relevance for practitioners. *Families in Society: The Journal of Contemporary Human Services, 76*(6), 395-407.

Freud, S. (1959). *Collected Papers* (Vol. 1) (Riviere, Trans.). New York: Basic Books.

Giorno, J. (1996). In P. Anderson (Ed.), *All of us: Americans talk about the meaning of death* (pp. 222-227). New York: Delacorte Press.

Granvold, D. (1996). Constructivist psychotherapy. *Families in Society: The Journal of Contemporary Human Services, 77*(6), 345-359.

Guba, E. (1990). *The paradigm dialog.* Newbury Park, CA: Sage Publications.

Kalish, R. (1980). *Death, grief and caring relationships.* Monterey, CA: Brooks/Cole.

Kastenbaum, R. (1975). Is death a crisis? On the confrontation with death in theory and practice. In N. Datan & L. Ginsberg (Eds.), *Life-span developmental psychology.* New York: Academic Press.

Keizer, B. (1994). *Dancing with Mister D.* New York: Doubleday.

Kelly, G. (1995). *The psychology of personal constructs.* New York: W. W. Norton.

Koenig, B., & Gates-Williams, J. (1995). Understanding cultural difference in caring for dying patients. In *Caring for Patients at the End of Life* [Special Issue]. *Western Journal of Medicine, 163,* 244-249.

Kornfield, J. (1993). *A path with heart.* New York: Bantam Books.

Maslow, A. (1985). *The farther reaches of human nature.* New York: Penguin Books.

Neimeyer, R., & Stewart, A. (1996). Trauma, healing, and the narrative employment of loss. *Families in Society: The Journal of Contemporary Human Services,* 360-375.

Peers, A. (Ed.). (Trans.). (1977). *Living flame of love: St. John of the Cross.* Linguori, MO: Triumph Books.

Sarbin, T. (1986). The narrative as a root metaphor for psychology. In T. R. Sarbin (Ed.), *Narrative psychology: The storied nature of human conduct* (pp. 3-21). New York: Praeger.

Smith, E. (1993). Spiritual awareness, personal perspective on death, and psychosocial distress among cancer patients: An initial investigation. *Journal of Psychosocial Oncology, 11*(3), 89-103.

Smith, E. (1995). Addressing the psychospiritual distress of death as reality: A transpersonal approach. *Social Work, 40*(3), 402-413.

Spiegel, M., & Tristman, R. (1997). *The grim reaper.* New York: Doubleday.

Walsh, R., & Vaughan, F. (1982). What is a person? *New Realities, 4*(6), 48-52.

Washburn, M. (1988). *The ego and the dynamic ground.* Albany: State University of New York Press.

Transpersonalism and Social Work Practice: Awakening to New Dimensions for Client Self-Determination, Empowerment, and Growth

Arlen Keith Leight

SUMMARY. This article proposes and advocates integration of a transpersonal model into clinical social work practice as a logical extension of the profession's inclusive perspective. The theory and practice of a transpersonal approach to psychotherapy and its applicability to social work are investigated, especially for use with marginalized populations. Transpersonalism is examined as an opportunity to enhance the worker's ability to respect and honor client self-determination, facilitate bio-psycho-social-spiritual growth and development, and empower even the most vulnerable in our society. *[Article copies available for a fee from The Haworth Document Delivery Service: 1-800-342-9678. E-mail address: <getinfo@haworthpressinc.com> Website: <http://www.Haworth Press.com> © 2001 by The Haworth Press, Inc. All rights reserved.]*

Arlen Keith Leight, DDS, MSW, is currently a practicing dentist and psychotherapist and lectures on clinical social work from a transpersonal perspective. Dr. Leight received psychotherapy training at American University in Washington, DC. He is co-founder with his mentor, Dr. Elizabeth Smith, of Transpersonal Psychotherapy of Washington in the nation's capital.

Address correspondence to: Arlen Keith Leight, DDS, MSW, Transpersonal Psychotherapy of Washington, Suite 714, 1145 19th Street, NW, Washington, DC 20036.

[Haworth co-indexing entry note]: "Transpersonalism and Social Work Practice: Awakening to New Dimensions for Client Self-Determination, Empowerment, and Growth." Leight, Arlen Keith. Co-published simultaneously in *Social Thought* (The Haworth Press, Inc.) Vol. 20, No. 1/2, 2001, pp. 63-76; and: *Transpersonal Perspectives on Spirituality in Social Work* (ed: Edward R. Canda, and Elizabeth D. Smith) The Haworth Press, Inc. 2001, pp. 63-76. Single or multiple copies of this article are available for a fee from The Haworth Document Delivery Service [1-800-342-9678, 9:00 a.m. - 5:00 p.m. (EST). E-mail address: getinfo@haworthpressinc.com].

KEYWORDS. Transpersonal, social work, empowerment, oppression, diversity

INTRODUCTION

The profession of social work has, at its core, a commitment and respect for the client as a whole entity seen in the context of the environment. The "big picture" approach to care sets the social worker apart from other mental health care professionals, many of whom focus solely on developmental and/or intrapsychic phenomena. Despite the expansive and inclusive nature of the social work perspective, there has been sparse attention paid to the human spiritual condition and dimensions beyond the ego. A transpersonal approach to client care encompasses realms of expanding consciousness, unitive social and spiritual connectedness, and human purpose and potentiality. A holistic model of practice is more comprehensive with the incorporation of the "phenomenological, the intuitive and the transpersonal" (Cowley, 1996, p. 668).

Social work, in its striving to be recognized as a serious and scientifically-based profession, often has been leery of an association with the unconventional, transpersonal perspective. The work of self-transcendence sometimes has been deemed inappropriate for clients whose basic life needs for food, shelter, and medical care have not been fulfilled. Recognizing social workers' traditional purpose as guardian of and advocate for the most vulnerable in our society, many in the field question the validity of work that is focused on those who are more fortunate (Cowley, 1996). While the continuing debate regarding the social worker's role is legitimate, a transpersonal model of practice may be appropriate for work with vulnerable clients and may offer the profession a valuable modality for clinical practice with oppressed and devalued populations.

Social work rightfully takes great pride in providing clients a broad biopsychosocial perspective. A transpersonal approach affords the worker added context, content, and process for addressing environmental, societal, and cultural stressors, non-pathologic transrational phenomena, and the grief associated with human existential suffering. As such, transpersonalism actually enhances and promotes respect for self-determination while empowering the client and facilitating bio-psycho-social-spiritual growth.

This article proposes and advocates integration of a transpersonal model into clinical social work practice as a logical extension of the profession's inclusive perspective. The definitions, the theory and the practice of a transpersonal approach to psychotherapy and its applicability to social work are investigated, especially for use with marginalized populations. We conclude by examining transpersonalism as an opportunity to enhance the worker's ability to respect and honor client self-determination, facilitate bio-psycho-social-spiritual growth and development, and empower even the most vulnerable in our society.

TRANSPERSONAL THEORY AND PRACTICE

Background

Transpersonal literally breaks down as "beyond/through" plus persona, meaning "mask" (Cowley, 1993, p. 527). Transpersonal, then, means beyond the person or beyond the ego. Transpersonalism is based on the assumption that there is a "higher or inner self distinct from the personal ego" (Guest, 1989, p. 63). Lajoie and Shapiro (1992) reviewed the first 23 years of transpersonal literature in search of a comprehensive definition of transpersonal psychology. The most frequently discovered themes in the 40 definitions cited include: (a) states of consciousness, (b) highest or ultimate potential, (c) beyond ego or personal self, (d) transcendence, and (e) spiritual. The authors propose a "contemporary definition" of transpersonal psychology: "Transpersonal psychology is concerned with the study of humanity's highest potential, and with the recognition, understanding and realization of intuitive, spiritual and transcendent states of consciousness" (p. 91).

Transpersonal psychology is based on a developmental perspective that acknowledges access to "higher" levels of being, to the "unitive self or Real Self" beyond the personal (Cowley, 1993, p. 527). Personal or personality development, in a psychotherapeutic context, is explained in terms of three "forces" of theory (Cowley, 1996): First Force (psychoanalytic), Second Force (behavioral), and Third Force (humanistic). The First Force deals with unconscious drives and impulses mainly from a pathological viewpoint. The Second Force, with its empirical focus, speaks to the process of socialization and learning theory. The Third Force is associated with humanistic, experiential and existential theory. Often associated with Abraham Maslow, Third Force self-actualization forms the philosophical basis for the Fourth Force of psychology which he described (as cited in Cowley, 1996) as "transpersonal, trans-human, centered in the cosmos rather than in human needs and interests, going beyond humanness, identity, self-actualization and the like" (p. 667).

Transpersonal psychology consists of a theoretical base and a practical base. While many theorists and practitioners appear in the literature, the prolific writings of Wilber and Washburn are generally associated with theory, and the work of Grof, Walsh, and Vaughan are generally associated with practice (Bynum, 1992). Walsh and Vaughan (1980) described transpersonal psychotherapy as a model of practice that includes traditional (first three Forces) areas and techniques. However, added to the mix is "an interest in facilitating growth and awareness beyond traditionally recognized levels of health. In so doing, the importance of modifying consciousness is emphasized, and the validity of transpersonal experience and identity is affirmed" (p. 9). Ken Wilber (as cited in Walsh & Vaughan, 1980) contended that if life is a dream, traditional psychotherapy is used to prevent the dream from becoming a nightmare, whereas transpersonal psychotherapy is used to facilitate awakening. Cowley (1993) suggests the use of a transpersonal approach with "clients whose problems or goals are spiritual in nature and who desire to transcend an exclusive identity with the ego" (p. 527).

Scotton (as cited in Hutton, 1994) described transpersonal psychotherapy as a modality that seeks to establish a "conscious and growth-producing link between the patient and the transpersonal experience." This includes an emphasis on the wholeness, the completion or the fruition which is to be found in the collective, transcendent or the spiritual" (p. 140).

Transpersonal practice involves an opening to higher stages of consciousness development. It is a "contemplative discovery" related to a "meditative or contemplative unfolding" (Wilber, 1997, p. 94). Wilber (1997) described three modes of knowing: (a) the eye of the flesh, associated with empiricism; (b) the eye of the mind, associated with rationalism; and (c) the eye of contemplation, associated with mysticism. All three modes are valid, but the nature of Spirit "can only be disclosed by the eye of contemplation" (p. 93). As such, the literature to date gives a theoretical, qualitative and contemplative look at transpersonal practice. This is reasonable given that knowledge regarding the essence of transpersonal phenomena is accessed through the eye of contemplation. The applicability of a rational positivist scientific formulation to the study of transpersonal experience may be untenable. That which is known by the eye of contemplation cannot be translated into the language of the eye of the flesh or the eye of the mind.

In summary, the literature defines transpersonal psychology as the study of experiences beyond the personal (Walsh & Vaughan, 1993). Transpersonal psychotherapy, then, holistically encompasses and "goes beyond existing models of practice to include self-transcendence . . . in shaping experience and enhancing well-being" (Walsh & Vaughan, 1980, p. 5). A transpersonal approach is an inclusive, holistic model of practice that enables the social work practitioner to provide clients a bio-psycho-social-spiritual framework for personal empowerment, development, and growth.

Theoretical Insights on Empowerment

Abraham Maslow, considered the father of both Humanistic (Third Force) and Transpersonal (Fourth Force) psychology, held (as cited by Vaughan, 1991) that human beings have innate spiritual needs and yearn for transcendent experiences. Ken Wilber (as cited by Vaughan, 1991) asserted that all drives are "subsets of the fundamental drive to attain unity with the Absolute" (p. 105). Accordingly, the healthiest people are thought to be those individuals who are able to incorporate spirituality into a sense of Self.

Psychological development, according to a transpersonal perspective, is viewed as a process in which "the whole of any level becomes a part of the whole of the next level" as consciousness evolves (Wilber, 1979, p. 2). Transpersonal theorists speak of three major developmental phases: prepersonal, personal, and transpersonal or preconventional, conventional, and transconventional. The first two levels are recognized, taught, nurtured, and expected by the society at large. The transpersonal or transconventional, on the other hand, is often seen as frightening and/or threatening to the individual and/or the society. Moving beyond the conventional requires a willingness to "relinquish attachments to social approval and the consensual world view" (Walsh, 1995, p. 350-351). As such, transpersonal development is often suppressed by a society that sees identification with an alternative belief system as a danger to the status quo.

An analogous dynamic is in operation with regard to marginalization and oppression in the society at large. The devalued individual's ability to develop his or her unique identity is thwarted by a threatened society. As such, the oppressor uses subtle strategies to suppress expression of an alternative belief system, lifestyle, or creative soulfulness. The oppressed, in attempting to reconcile internal truth with external pressures, are, as such, propitiously positioned and inherently inclined to relinquish attachment to a world view that creates intense personal discord and disharmony. Such a willingness is central to the proposition that a transpersonal approach provides a perspective, not an escape, for propelling growth and empowerment in oppressed social work clients.

The first Noble Truth in Buddhism identifies the inherent suffering that exists in the manifest world. Transpersonal perspectives center on identity and alienation. Suffering is recognized as a case of "mistaken identity" (Walsh, 1995, p. 347). Self-alienation results from our defensive posture or "defensively contracted state" (Walsh & Vaughan, 1980, p. 10) as we try to squeeze our true selves into a conditioned, conventional, societal mold or world view. A "self-masking" ensues which we do not normally recognize because "we have been hypnotized since infancy, we actively defend it, we all share in it, and because we live in the biggest cult of all: culture" (Walsh, 1995, p. 349).

Society functions by both creating a fictitious reality to which we unwittingly succumb and by preventing awareness of reality to which we innately aspire (Walsh & Vaughan, 1980). We are seduced into the conventional lifestyle and live in a trance-like state consisting of developmental stagnation with its accompanying existential suffering. Uncontrollable thoughts, busyness, materialism and preoccupation with the details of day-to-day living keep us bound and attached to a limited view of ourselves within our environmental circumstances (Walsh, 1995). As espoused in the second and third Noble Truths of Buddhism, since attachment is at the core of our suffering, letting go is at the core of its cessation. Transpersonalism provides a context for letting go, for transcending this egoistic state of consciousness, for moving beyond preoccupation with self, and moving toward (or back to) a connection with the whole.

Oppressed and devalued clients are often most vulnerable to self-alienation. A damaging denial of the true self is reinforced by the oppressors who perpetually strive to maintain status quo control. Whether working with the oppressed or the oppressor, the social worker does well to understand that the source of the suffering is the unacknowledged clinging to the defensively contracted state.

Defensive contraction can be relaxed by "quieting the mind and reducing perceptual distortion" (Walsh & Vaughan, 1980, p. 11). Ram Dass (as cited in Walsh & Vaughan, 1980) stated, "We are all prisoners of our minds. This realization is the first step in the journey of freedom" (p. 11). The goals of transpersonal therapy include "the extinction of awareness from this conditioned tyranny of the mind" (Walsh & Vaughan, 1980, p. 12) and the movement "to a state beyond identification" (Smith, 1995, p. 406).

Transpersonal approaches see a healthy process as one that dis-identifies from conditioned consciousness in order to transcend ego attachments. The basic concept, as stated by Assagioli (as cited in Walsh & Vaughan, 1980), is that "we are dominated by everything with which our self becomes identified. We can dominate and control everything from which we dis-identify" (p. 14). Without identification there is no suffering. Marginalized clients may indeed benefit from a dis-identification from the negative beliefs and induced feelings attributed to them by the oppressive, dominant culture which are subsequently internalized as mistaken identity. It must be noted, however, that a transpersonal approach does not advocate evading materiality. As Mark Epstein (1995) explained, "All of the insults to our narcissism can be overcome, the Buddha proclaimed, not by escaping them, but by uprooting the conviction in a 'self' that needs protecting" (p. 45). The transpersonal approach affords the worker an effective and potent social work model for empowering the client to move beyond the suffering, beyond the false self to an identity that feels truly genuine and honest.

The theoretical foundation of transpersonalism identifies an awakening process in which the defensively contracted state is relinquished by progressive disidentification, guided by the eye of contemplation, leading to a state of pure awareness. One is ultimately nothing and everything, nowhere and everywhere, in time and outside of time. A state of bliss ensues as there is no attachment, and, therefore, no suffering (Walsh & Vaughan, 1980). Unity with the Absolute is finally achieved.

A Transpersonal Approach to Practice

Transpersonal psychotherapy, in keeping with a philosophically based inclusive stance, incorporates the conventional psychodynamic process as well as the traditional goals of symptom reduction and behavioral modification. The transpersonal psychotherapist additionally "aims to assist the client in disidentifying from and transcending psychodynamic issues" (Walsh & Vaughan, 1980, p. 18). Transpersonal psychotherapy is significantly influenced by Eastern thought as it is blended with traditional Western approaches. Classical psychoanalysis (First Force) seeks to strengthen the ego while transpersonal therapy seeks to help the client discover the true self by disidentification from the ego. Behaviorism (Second Force) seeks "cognitive mediation of behavior" while transpersonal therapy uses techniques such as meditation and visualization often "viewed from within a behavioral modification framework." Humanistic psychotherapy (Third Force) values self-actualization while transpersonal psychotherapy incorporates a "capacity for self-transcendence beyond self-actualization" (Walsh & Vaughan, 1980, pp. 24-25).

For example, in a clinical situation, a gay client coming out in mid-life may present with feelings of confusion, anger, grief, and guilt. Walsh and Vaughan (1980) explained that the psychodynamic therapist would be interested in history and ego assessment and would try to determine the origins of the thoughts causing the negative feelings. The behaviorist might examine ways to change the thoughts through a cognitive or learning process. The humanistic therapist might work with the client to understand sexual fulfillment in the context of self-actualization. The transpersonal therapist may well incorporate the same approaches but would also work on the client's identification with the negative thoughts and feelings. Techniques such as meditation and visualization may be utilized to help the client disidentify from those negative thoughts and feelings and move beyond the defensively contracted state.

Michael Hutton (1994) conducted a survey of transpersonal psychotherapists to determine how they differ from traditional therapists both in therapeutic technique and personal beliefs and practices. Transpersonal practitioners agree with traditional practitioners that all psychotherapists need to be grounded in traditional theories of psychotherapy. However, unlike transpersonalists, traditional therapists generally feel that spiritual interests have little or nothing to do with psychotherapy. Ninety-two percent of the transpersonal therapists reported experiencing or possibly experiencing a spiritual force which seemed to lift them outside themselves, while 79% of psychoanalysts and 55% of behavioral/cognitive therapists had not. As well, the transpersonal therapists generally performed some personal spiritual practice two to three times per day, including prayer, meditation, or spiritual reading. In terms of techniques, transpersonal therapists utilized intuition, meditation, relaxation, visualization, spiritual focus, spiritual and religious writings, and dreamwork significantly more often than traditional practitioners.

Scotton (as cited in Hutton, 1994) asserted that transpersonal psychotherapists need to have a firm grounding in traditional psychotherapy, need to be open to and have knowledge regarding a variety of spiritual paths, and need to be actively pursuing a personal path of spiritual development. As such, social workers can feel assured about a transpersonal practice model that includes and enhances traditional psychotherapeutic techniques, acknowledges and respects a client's spiritual pursuits, encourages and honors the worker's spiritual path, and facilitates and expedites human growth and development.

A Transpersonal Framework for Empowerment-Oriented Practice

Au-Deane Cowley (1996) proposed "Transpersonal Practice" as a social work model to deal with "client systems at every level on the Full Spectrum of Consciousness" (p. 680). This comprehensive approach includes work on six different dimensions: physical, emotional, cognitive, psychosocial, moral, and spiritual. Assessment and treatment of the client's distress across all dimensions creates a mind-body-spirit approach. Contextual variables include family and relationships, social institutions, physical environment, cultural factors, gender issues, economic situations, historical factors, and macro systems. Key concepts include connectedness of the contextual variables, encompassing the holistic flavor of a transpersonal approach. All Four Forces of theory (i.e., psychoanalytic, behavioral, humanistic, and transpersonal) are available for use in this model.

Elizabeth Smith (1995) described a "Transegoic Model" in which a four stage approach for dealing with the psychospiritual distress of death is delineated. These stages include ego disattachment and self-transcendence in which a disidentification from the ego "empowers the client to assign new meaning to the image of self," and definitions of the transpersonal self and the transpersonal mission are established. The future is thus envisioned in a new context as "the worker helps the client identify and work from a place of love rather than fear" (p. 409).

Expanded use of transpersonalism in social work practice may grow out of an understanding of the context, content, and process of transpersonal psychotherapy (Vaughan, 1979). Transpersonal context, as illustrated in both the Cowley and Smith practice models, refers to the openness, mutuality, and love which form the basis of an arena for change. The atmosphere or tone of the therapy is "determined entirely by the beliefs, values, and intentions of the therapist." This transpersonal context helps to remove obstacles to "transpersonal awakening or personal transformation." "If the therapist does not believe such change is possible, disbelief becomes an obstacle" (p. 104). As such, transpersonal context supports the basic tenets of social work practice, i.e., starting where the client is, respecting client self-determination, and honoring the client's perspective.

Three hypothetical examples may help to illustrate the importance of transpersonal context:

1. A 63-year-old Caucasian man presents himself to you as an incest survivor now dealing with the death of his father. He explains that he believes he existed as spirit prior to his incarnation on the planet, and, at that time, chose the two people he felt would make ideal parents for working on his issues in this lifetime. In essence, he tells you he chose his incestuous father.
2. A 40-year-old Hispanic woman relates she was about to die from AIDS when she discovered an ancient meditation involving the creation of a primordial sound. After demonstrating the technique, she explains she is now well and HIV negative, but she feels guilty about and mourns the loss of her husband who recently died of AIDS.
3. A 27-year-old African American graduate student presents with problems in establishing and maintaining intimate relationships. She explains that 2 or 3 times per week at 4:00 in the morning she leaves her body to explore other countries and planets.

The experiences of these individuals are "transrational" or beyond reason as we normally assess clients in our conventional paradigms. Traditional psychotherapy is pathology based, and, therefore, our first inclination is to think pathology. "In fact, Freud's collected works contain over 400 references to neurosis and none to health" (Walsh & Vaughan, 1980, p. 7). A transpersonal context requires a paradigm shift to recognize and understand that some nonrational experiences are transpersonal phenomena and not necessarily pathologic in nature.

The social worker limited to a First, Second and/or Third Force model of practice would likely never encounter these extraordinarily personal and transrational accounts. Unless the worker's context is open to such realms, client's fears about being misunderstood or disrespected might prevent complete disclosure. However, if a worker were to be confronted with such a transrational client history without the benefit of a transpersonal context, grand opportunities for personal transformation and growth may be lost. Starting where the client is and respecting the client's perspective and self-determination necessarily require the social worker to consider the possibility of a transpersonal experience. The transpersonal context does not negate the possibility of pathology but rather necessitates an assessment of the transrational. It is possible that the 63-year-old incest survivor comes from an Eastern or Buddhist perspective. The 40-year-old client may indeed be one of the rare seroconverters and can present medical records documenting a change from HIV+ to HIV−. The 27-year-old student may have discovered lucid dreaming, a well documented phenomenon characterized as the ability to take conscious awareness into the dream state. Once pathology is ruled out, transpersonal context can "facilitate the exploration of transpersonal content," and, as such, the client's transrational experience can be used by the worker to facilitate growth and change (Vaughan, 1979, p. 104).

"Transpersonal content refers to any experience in which an individual transcends the limitations of identifying exclusively with the ego or personality" (Vaughan, 1979, p. 104). Transpersonal content encompasses the discussion of "paranormal" and/or spiritual phenomena (Boorstein, 1986, p. 123). Such experiences are not valued as the goal of therapy but rather as potential resources for growth and empowerment. As such, transpersonal phenomena are "useful in facilitating disidentification from superficial roles and distorted self-image" (Vaughan, 1979, p. 105). These superficial roles and distorted self-images are often a major source of suffering in oppressed clients. Gays and lesbians, African Americans, and the homeless are often marginalized against their will and labeled in a cruel and dehumanizing manner resulting in significant spiritual distress. "Being marginal to society can be an opportunity" to work with an approach that "transcends culture and ego" (Struzzo, 1989, p. 204). As such, social workers can broaden their scope of practice with vulnerable clients by utilizing and working with any disclosed transpersonal content. The therapist is not required to agree with any particular belief system or validate any particular experience but rather does well to incorporate the transpersonal content into "the full spectrum of the client's life experience" (Vaughan, 1979, p. 105).

For example, Ronald Wang Jue (1988) used regression therapy as a transpersonal modality with a 32-year-old hermaphrodite who was raised to be female but decided to assume an adult male identity. Regression therapy utilizing hypnosis helped the client to recall past-life memories which focused on a choice of sexual orientation. The transpersonal therapist did not treat the memories as historical truth, but rather remained open to the client's reality or "felt-truths" (p. 7) as a context for therapy. The transrational experiences in the hypnotic state provided the transpersonal content that helped the client to go beyond the societal expectations that were the basis for distress. Disidentification from the ego and the defensively contracted state brought the client to a place of self-empowerment and self-acceptance. Social work's commitment to empowering the devalued and marginalized individual was thereby supported and enhanced.

The progression illustrated in this clinical case exemplifies transpersonal process. Transpersonal process, while nonlinear, recognizes an identification stage "concerned with developing ego strength, raising self-esteem and letting go of negative patterns of self-invalidation" as is normally associated with traditional (first three Forces) therapeutic techniques (Vaughan, 1979, p. 105). A disidentification stage involves "transpersonal awakening" in which "the self is experienced as an independent entity" free from meaningless worldly attachments (Vaughan, 1979, p. 105). Suffering that seems insoluble at the ego level is ultimately transcended.

John A. Struzzo (1989), in discussing a transpersonal process for gays and lesbians, pointed out that "ego centered psychotherapy tends to focus on adaptation to one's culture" (p. 204). Inasmuch as the culture is inherently homophobic and heterosexist, such adaptation is clearly unhealthy for homosexual clients. Assisting gays and lesbians "to disidentify from the restrictions of their personality, and to realize their identity with their total [real] self" offers a more viable alternative for growth and empowerment (p. 201).

Molefi Kete Asante (1984) explained that "rhythm is a principle path to transcendence for African Americans" (p. 177). The transpersonal process involves "joining in the collective expression of power" (p. 172). A "search for harmony" beyond the individual, beyond the self, beyond the ego is "at the base of African American spirituality" (p. 175). Social work with African American clients benefits from an understanding of empowerment potentially attainable through such a significant transpersonal process.

Carol Montgomery (1994) interviewed women who had overcome homelessness and discovered that personal, interpersonal, and transpersonal strengths influenced growth toward personal empowerment. The homelessness and hard times created a context for a transpersonal process in which a "new self" developed allowing the women to transcend "the chaos of their individual lives and . . . make peace with what had happened to them." One woman said she "was forced to find goodness within herself." Another explained, "Like a caterpillar . . . I became a beautiful, beautiful butterfly" (p. 42-43). A transpersonal process empowered these homeless women to make a self-determined choice to move beyond a limited view of self and toward a loving space for growth and change.

CONCLUSIONS

The transpersonal model of practice fits well within the parameters of the social work perspective. The client's societal context and its effect on the individual's perception of self is integral to both transpersonal psychotherapy and social work. Providing a loving space and being open to the client's perspective are fundamental to both schools of practice. A transpersonal experience, moving toward higher levels of consciousness, awakens both a sense of wholeness and connectedness essential to the social responsiveness that is at the heart of social work's mission (Cowley, 1996). "Compassion, generosity, inner peace and the capacity for relatedness in the world . . . tend to be manifested as a result of transpersonal work" (Vaughan, 1979, p. 108). Cowley (1996) came to the determination that a transpersonal approach, "By acknowledging the important contributions of all major psychological theories, and by taking into account and validating the transrational nature of the spiritual dimension, the artificial divisions and omissions in clinical practice can be healed or made whole" (p. 694).

The context, content, and process of a transpersonal approach offer social work practitioners expanded opportunity for empowering oppressed and vulnerable clients. Self-determination is honored as bio-psycho-social-spiritual growth enhanced through this model of practice. Social work, with its inclusive perspective, its openness and respect for diversity and difference, and its responsibility for and responsiveness to the individual and to the society, is positioned as the most available profession to be at the forefront of a movement and model of transpersonal practice that promotes human liberation, growth, and interconnectedness.

Yet Fourth Force psychotherapy as a model of practice for social work is in its infancy (Cowley, 1996). Aside from Smith's work with the terminally ill and scattered work with substance abusers, there is little population-specific research. Social work, in particular, needs to examine transpersonal practice with vulnerable clients. Those marginalized by society may be the most readily able to benefit from a transpersonal approach.

Transpersonalism has the unfortunate distinction of being associated with New Age gurus and pop psychology (Taylor, 1992). Spiritual in nature, the model tends to create fear in the hearts of the scientist-social worker who has been striving for years to gain recognition and secure respectful status in the community of professionals. However, as our Western culture opens to Eastern philosophical thought in the context of post modernism, social work can benefit by opening to the potential applications of a transpersonal, bio-psycho-social-spiritual approach that recognizes the status of the human condition in the societal context and works to alleviate existential suffering and dis-ease of the spiritual dimension.

REFERENCES

Asante, M. K. (1984). The African American mode of transcendence. *The Journal of Transpersonal Psychology, 16,* 167-177.

Boorstein, S. (1986). Transpersonal context, interpretation and psychotherapeutic technique. *The Journal of Transpersonal Psychology, 18,* 123-130.

Bynum, E. B. (1992). A brief overview of transpersonal psychology. *The Humanistic Psychologist, 20,* 301-306.

Cowley, A. S. (1993). Transpersonal social work: A theory for the 1990's. *Social Work, 38,* 527-534.

Cowley, A. S. (1996). Transpersonal social work. In F. J. Turner (Ed.), *Social work treatment: Interlocking theoretical approaches* (4th ed., pp. 663-698). New York: The Free Press.

Epstein, M. (1995). *Thoughts without a thinker.* New York: Basic Books.

Guest, H. (1989). The origins of transpersonal psychology. *British Journal of Psychotherapy, 6,* 62-69.

Hutton, M. S. (1994). How transpersonal psychotherapists differ from other practitioners: An empirical study. *The Journal of Transpersonal Psychology, 26,* 139-174.

Jue, R. W. (1988). Regression therapy as a transpersonal modality. *The Journal of Transpersonal Psychology, 20,* 4-9.

Lajoie, D. H., & Shapiro, S. I. (1992). Definitions of transpersonal psychology: The first twenty-three years. *The Journal of Transpersonal Psychology, 24,* 79-98.

Montgomery, C. (1994). Swimming upstream: The strengths of women who survive homelessness. *Advances in Nursing Science, 16,* 34-45.

Smith, E. D. (1995). Addressing the psychospiritual distress of death as reality: A transpersonal approach. *Social Work, 40,* 402-413.

Struzzo, J. A. (1989). Pastoral counseling and homosexuality. *Journal of Homosexuality, 18,* 195-222.

Taylor, E. (1992). Transpersonal psychology: Its several virtues. *The Humanistic Psychologist, 20,* 285-300.

Vaughan, F. (1979). Transpersonal psychotherapy: Context, content, process. *The Journal of Transpersonal Psychology, 11,* 101-128.

Vaughan, F. (1991). Spiritual issues in psychotherapy. *The Journal of Transpersonal Psychology, 23,* 105-119.

Walsh, R. (1995). The problem of suffering: Existential and transpersonal perspectives. *The Humanistic Psychologist, 23,* 345-357.

Walsh, R., & Vaughan, F. (1980). Beyond the ego: Toward transpersonal models of the person and psychotherapy. *Journal of Humanistic Psychology, 20,* 5-31.

Walsh, R., & Vaughan, F. (1993). On transpersonal definitions. *The Journal of Transpersonal Psychology, 25,* 199-207.

Wilber, K. (1979). A developmental view of consciousness. *The Journal of Transpersonal Psychology, 11,* 1-21.

Wilber, K. (1997). Transpersonal hot spots: Reflections on the new editions of *Up from Eden, the Atman Project,* and *Eye to Eye. Journal of Humanistic Psychology, 37,* 74-103.

Cosmic Consciousness: Path or Pathology?

Au-Deane S. Cowley

SUMMARY. Historically the relationship between spirituality and mental health has been characterized by confusion in terms of what constitutes healthy spirituality (path) as opposed to psychotic states (pathology). Finding criteria to help differentiate *pre*-rational structures from *trans*-rational structures (since they are both *non*-rational) has been an elusive goal. Ken Wilber's Full Spectrum of Consciousness Model, presented in 1986, is the only transpersonal theory that offers descriptors for three general levels of consciousness (prepersonal, personal, and transpersonal), the pathologies likely to develop at each level of development, as well as preferred interventions for developmental problems at each level of consciousness. This chapter applies Wilber's model and related ideas from other transpersonal theorists in order to provide differential assessment guidelines for therapists working with the spiritual dimension of clients' experience. *[Article copies available for a fee from The Haworth Document Delivery Service: 1-800-342-9678. E-mail address: <getinfo@haworthpressinc.com> Website: <http://www.Haworth Press.com> © 2001 by The Haworth Press, Inc. All rights reserved.]*

KEYWORDS. Transpersonal practice, spiritual pathologies, path or healthy spirituality, pre-trans fallacy, Full Spectrum of Consciousness, mental health, assessment

---

Address correspondence to: Au-Deane S. Cowley, PhD, Professor Emerita, 478 No. Pinion Hills Drive, Dammeron Valley, UT 84783 (Email: adcowley@earthlink.net).

[Haworth co-indexing entry note]: "Cosmic Consciousness: Path or Pathology?" Cowley, Au-Deane S. Co-published simultaneously in *Social Thought* (The Haworth Press, Inc.) Vol. 20, No. 1/2, 2001, pp. 77-94; and: *Transpersonal Perspectives on Spirituality in Social Work* (ed: Edward R. Canda, and Elizabeth D. Smith) The Haworth Press, Inc. 2001, pp. 77-94. Single or multiple copies of this article are available for a fee from The Haworth Document Delivery Service [1-800-342-9678, 9:00 a.m. - 5:00 p.m. (EST). E-mail address: getinfo@haworthpressinc.com].

INTRODUCTION

Historically, the relationship between spirituality and mental health has been wildly erratic, ranging across a continuum of polar opposites. On one end of the continuum, Marx (1906) decried religion as the opiate of the people, and Freud (1946) viewed religiosity and mental illness as virtually synonymous. On the other end of the continuum, Jung viewed neurosis as the suffering of a soul which had not discovered its meaning (Campbell, 1971), and Emanuel Swedenborg (1872) postulated that human life depends on the relationship a person has to a hierarchy of spirits. In the 1990s, the helping professions landed somewhere between the polarized positions described on the continuum above.

Over the last two decades, professionals have increasingly taken a stand in terms of recognizing the importance of religious convictions and spiritual values in clinical social work practice (Brothers, 1992; Canda, 1988a, 1988b, 1989; Canda & Furman, 1999; Cowley, 1993, 1996a, 1996b, 1999; Derezotes, 2000; Joseph, 1987; Robbins, Chatterjee, & Canda, 1998; Russel, 1998; Sheridan, Bullis, Adcock, Berlin, & Miller, 1992). However, it seems that some educators and mental health workers in the post-modern age remain confused about whether they can come out of the closet and deal with issues related to religion, spirituality, mysticism, and the like without somehow undermining their professional respectability and/or credibility. To be "safe," some practitioners have chosen a path of avoidance. In making a plea for all kinds of helping professionals to become more sophisticated in religious and spiritual matters, M. Scott Peck (1978) wrote:

> Psychiatrists and psychotherapists that have simplistic attitudes toward religion are likely to do a disservice to some of their patients. This will be true if they regard all religion as good or healthy. It will also be true if they throw out the baby with the bath water and regard all religion as sickness or the Enemy. And, finally, it will be true if in the face of the complexity of the matter they withdraw themselves from dealing at all with the religious issues of their patients, hiding behind a cloak of such total objectivity that they do not consider it to be their role to be, themselves, in any way spiritually or religiously involved. For their patients often need their involvement. (p. 225)

Therapists, whether they intend to or not, often function in the uncomfortable but unavoidable role of secular priest (London, 1986, p. xii). Whether it is explicitly acknowledged or not, interventions ultimately involve the value dimensions of both therapist and client.

Psychotherapy is a moral force, and psychotherapists, in turn, are moral agents as well as healing technicians. Moral problems affect how therapists see their client's needs, set goals of treatment, and work in sessions. The fact is inherent in the enterprise. A century before Freud launched modern psychotherapy, Phillipe Pinel had named his psychiatric methods "moral treatment." (London, 1986, p. 1)

For most mental health practitioners, the prospect of needing to function as a moral agent to ameliorate problems in the spiritual dimension will require learning more about Fourth Force transpersonal theory.

Importance of the Spiritual Dimension

Over the last 30 years, clients have increasingly presented with problems related to spiritual practice and the spiritual dimension. In one Virginia study of 528 licensed professional counselors, clinical social workers, and psychologists, respondents reported that "religious issues played a role in about one-third of their client's current difficulties" (Bullis, 1996, p. 14). An area of practice that heretofore had been basically neglected (Joseph, 1987) could no longer be ignored. Looking for answers to spiritual questions took many practitioners for the first time into transpersonal literature and nontraditional ways of working with spiritual concerns.

In 1996, Boorstein asserted that transpersonal techniques and psychotherapy could be effectively utilized across the spectrum of consciousness and could even "heal and consolidate the ego at more fragile levels of psychological development" (p. 282). Such claims challenged therapists to explore and incorporate transpersonal approaches into their practice repertoire. In fact, some writers in the late eighties took the position that unless the spiritual aspect of clients is recognized, therapists not only fail to serve their clients well–but may also do irreparable harm (Canda, 1989; Grof & Grof, 1989; Hendlin, 1985).

Once the transpersonal approach was recognized as the Fourth Force of psychology, articles on the topic began to appear in social work literature. Increasingly, practitioners have begun to weave transpersonal theories not only into their clinical approaches but also into social policy decisions (Canda & Chambers, 1994; Derezotes, 2000). In terms of human growth and behavior, assessment of the person-in-environment context has become more likely to include the spiritual dimension as an integral aspect of healthy human development (Anthony, Ecker, & Wilber, 1987; Robbins, Chatterjee, & Canda, 1998). As Peay (1997) pointed out, illness or emotional problems are much more likely now to be seen as a reflection of the difficulties that coexist between a person and the larger world–including the spiritual elements involved in the equation (p. 34). Frankl's existential logotherapy of the late sixties was a precursor to the transpersonal social work of the late nineties. He wrote that a "proper diagnosis can be made only by someone who can see the spiritual side of man" (1968, p. ix).

Despite a growing tendency to include issues related to religion or spirituality into social work education and practice, until the last few years there has been little academic training offered in graduate social work programs to prepare practitioners for dealing with content related to the spiritual dimension (Canda, 1988a, 1989; Cowley, 1996a; Cowley, 1993; Cowley & Derezotes, 1994; Derezotes, 2000.) Thus, most social workers (and other helping professionals) have been generally ill-prepared to deal with such common religious problems as the loss or questioning of one's faith, a change in denominational membership, or the stress to the entire family system when a member becomes involved with a cult (Lukoff, Lu, & Turner, 1996). A national survey of 2,069 social workers involved in direct practice found that 73% had not received content on religion or spirituality in their graduate programs (Canda & Furman, 1999, p. 73). Other gaps in the preparation of practitioners include the absence of a theoretical foundation and/or specific intervention techniques for dealing with the problems that may unexpectedly accompany spiritually focused seminars or individual spiritual practice.

Grof and Grof (1989) coined the term "spiritual emergency" to describe recognizable spiritual maladies. Other practitioners have also acknowledged the practice challenges inherent in working with problems in the spiritual dimension:

> These problems present with intensities ranging from a mild form of "spiritual emergence" (a gradual unfoldment of spiritual potential with no disruption in psychological-social-occupation functioning) to a severe form of "spiritual emergency" (an uncontrolled emergence of spiritual phenomena with significant disruption in psychological-social-occupational functioning. (Lukoff, Lu, & Turner, 1996, p. 238)

In response, spiritual emergency networks and hotlines have been established in many localities around the country to deal with an exploding number of spiritually related issues and problems.

Viewing the Trans-Rational as Irrational

Due to the possibility of significant disruption of functioning occurring concomitantly with spiritual emergencies or mystical experiences, there has been a proclivity among mental health professionals to mistakenly view mystical experiences as psychotic episodes. The mistake involves confusion about trans-rational elements that emerge in the course of therapeutic sessions. Practitioners in many settings have probably echoed the question posed by Bucke in 1923: "How then shall we know that this (cosmic consciousness experience) is a new sense, revealing fact, and not a form of insanity, plunging its subject into delusion?" (p. 70).

Since some delusions may have features similar to religious experiences, it is easy to see how the two widely disparate states could be seen as one and the same. Both religious delusions and religious experiences may contain false beliefs, which an individual will vigorously defend, despite their logical absurdity, or even against proof to the contrary. Psychotic delusions assume many forms of expression and vary from the disjointed word salad of a person with schizophrenia to the logically consistent, delusional system of a person exhibiting a paranoid personality disorder. Furthermore, unbalanced religiosity can develop into a fanaticism that manifests with delusional features. No wonder this similarity between the non-rational and the irrational has often left the practitioner hard-pressed to distinguish pathological spirituality from other mental disturbances. It remained the task of transpersonal psychology to explicate the difference between the irrational (pre-personal), the rational (personal), and the trans-rational (transpersonal) levels of consciousness (Wilber, 1986):

> Because the personal level [of consciousness] has been viewed as the acme of human development by most Western schools of psychology, a recurrent trap has been to dismiss or pathologize transpersonal levels. Indeed, because some transpersonal experiences such as the dissolution of ego boundaries bear a superficial resemblance to some pathological conditions, there has been a tendency to equate the two. For example, mystical experiences have been interpreted as regressions to union with the breast, ecstatic states viewed as narcissistic neurosis, enlightenment dismissed as regression to intrauterine stages, and meditation seen as self-induced catatonia. This is the trap that Wilber calls the pre-trans fallacy. (Walsh & Vaughan, 1996, p. 63)

Widely publicized destructive acts by religious zealots added to the cultural lore connecting spirit with pathology and strengthened the tendency to confuse the two. Likewise, when people experience bad trips and a temporary collapse of ego instead of "enlightenment" while experimenting with mind altering drugs, it adds credence to the almost automatic connection some have made between "higher states of consciousness" and the somehow "flaky" or weird.

Since Wilber's theories and concepts are not widely integrated into the practice wisdom of the helping professions, many practitioners still do not have a knowledge base that could prepare them to avoid making a pre-trans fallacy. During assessment of a spiritual emergency, one might confuse *pre*-rational structures with *trans*-rational structures simply because both are *non*-rational (Wilber 1980; Wilber, 1986, p. 146).

PATH OR PATHOLOGY?

James's (1961) groundbreaking work early in the 1900s provided information about the varieties of religious experience. Today, professional helpers are increasingly coming to understand that each person develops a truly idiosyncratic way of expressing his/her spirituality. For some, religion may become a path–for others a pathology. As Vaughan (1995) so sagely observed, "Every tradition offers comforting illusions for those who would escape from freedom and roadmaps to liberation for those who choose to follow them" (p. 45). Welwood (1986a) agreed that there are vast variations that can occur as humans interact with religious and societal institutions out of their own unique spiritual potentialities. This complex interaction between environment, being, and spirit defies attempts to identify general predictors by which to understand the spiritual experiences of individual client-systems. If religious experience is anything, it is, at heart, a personal experience (Cowley, 1996b):

> There is no fixed prescription for how to be human. Unlike other animals, our nature is not defined by a repetitive daily round of fixed action patterns and survival routines. . . . Our nature is open-ended, malleable, never fully defined. (Welwood, 1986a, pp. 133-134)

Liester (1996) offered one creative way to distinguish between path and pathology when he suggested that there is a developmental hierarchy that helps one to differentiate between inner voices that are pathological and inner voices of a transcendent nature. "Lower level" or pathological inner voices are those voices that are regressive or prepersonal. They include hallucinations, pseudohallucinations, and illusions. Healthy, transcendent or transpersonal voices are "higher" up the developmental hierarchy (higher states of consciousness) and range "upward" from imagination to intuition to revelation (p. 5).

Since "the nature of consciousness changes the nature of reality" (Bullis, 1996, p. 106), learning how to discriminate helpful from harmful inner voices and authentic from regressive spiritual practices is one of the prime challenges that cultural pluralism poses to individuals and practitioners alike (Anthony,

Ecker, & Wilber, 1987). Cults and mind-warping collectives abound in the 21st century and apparently provide tempting lures to those seeking a spiritual home and a sense of community. Sometimes this search for "security" leads spiritual seekers down dangerous and even fatal paths. To serve their clients well, practitioners need to be prepared to help them discriminate between an authentic path and one that is potentially regressive:

> What is spiritual authenticity and how can we distinguish it from shallow, pseudomystical rationalizations of self-interest? How can we recognize signs of psychological pathology in a group or leader, and so avoid involvements that maintain and even exaggerate members' psychopathology under the guise of higher development. (Anthony, Ecker, & Wilber, 1987, p. 2)

The practice dilemma of discerning whether a person or group is operating out of higher consciousness or is pathologically disturbed may be further complicated by the fact that it is so rare for individuals to reach the farther limits of human potential that very little information exists about these states of consciousness (Wilber, 1999). Additionally, literature dealing with transpersonal theory and the spiritual dimension is not often included in mainstream professional journals. Thus, this information is not widely accessible to mental health workers. This means that comparatively few practitioners are qualified to understand the spiritual plights of their clients.

A therapist may feel intimidated when approached by a client who is struggling with issues of ultimate concerns and deeply held values. If one is not conversant with the belief system of the client or transpersonal therapies, referral ought to be considered. When working with the spiritual dimension, one skill that is essential is to keep one's own belief systems out of the way while helping the client to find his/her own answers. In seeking to clarify who is conceptually qualified to deal with issues related to the transpersonal or spiritual dimension, Walsh and Vaughan (1980) posited two relevant philosophical concepts. These two concepts are: *adequatio,* which states that the understanding of the knower must be adequate to the thing to be known, and *grades of significance,* which points out that the same phenomenon may hold entirely different grades of meaning and significance to different observers with different degrees of adequatio" (p. 45). As Wade (1996) has also posited:

> Understanding a higher level of awareness is not fully possible by people at lower levels, especially the ineffability of the Unity level. In fact, the propensity for misunderstanding is so great that it is the primary reason mystical teachings have been restricted to qualified initiates rather than broadcast. (p. 210)

If practitioners are going to meet the practice challenges of the 21st century, they can no longer remain among the uninitiated when it comes to understanding what encourages and what inhibits the development of human potential in terms of spirituality and higher levels of consciousness.

A pioneering endeavor to articulate the differences between higher states of consciousness and psychotic experiencing occurred in the early 1900s, more than a half-century before the birth of the transpersonal movement. In a classic study of the evolution of the human mind, Bucke (1923) provided early descriptions of cosmic consciousness. Bucke held that consciousness is a human potential which, when evolved in the human species, allows individuals to grasp the meaning of human existence in relation to the cosmos (West, 1985). He posited that when an individual transcended the self to experience cosmic consciousness, it was an indication of optimum spiritual health. In retrospect, Bucke's work was probably an idea whose time had not yet come. His leading edge work received little or no attention from professional educators or practitioners in mental health fields. Bucke was, nonetheless, one of the first scholars to try to describe the characteristics of cosmic consciousness. He was also one of the first to question how we might contrast those having cosmic consciousness experiences to profiles of those who had psychosis.

Buck suggested three considerations to help distinguish whether a person is experiencing higher states of consciousness or a pathological episode: (1) *The previous character and attributes of the individual.* If a person has had a consistent work history as well as long term reciprocal relationships, it is less likely that a religious or mystical experience is a psychotic one. Conversely, if the person has been a long-term patient under psychiatric care or has a history of failed relationships as well as a poorly integrated work identity, the likelihood that he/she is experiencing a psychotic process rather than illumination is greatly increased; (2) *Age at onset.* In Bucke's view, people generally do not have cosmic or higher consciousness experiences prior to mid-life; (3) *The experience of a sudden awakening.* Bucke said that cosmic consciousness often arises suddenly with experiences of spiritual illumination and visions of white light.

To find more recently developed criteria that will help us distinguish between healthy and pathological spirituality, we must turn to the emerging body of transpersonal theory since it is the only major psychological theory that focuses on the spiritual dimension. Current descriptors of transrational states coming out of transpersonal studies differ somewhat from Bucke's earlier conceptions. History of personal development is still viewed by most Fourth Force writers as an important consideration, but transpersonalists are more likely to focus on developmental gains that have accrued over time due to sustained spiritual practice than they are on "sudden awakenings" (Bloomfield, 1980;

Walsh & Vaughan, 1993). Transpersonal literature is more likely to view peak experiences as transformative states that can occur at any level of consciousness. Thus, age or isolated illuminating incidents are less likely to be seen as evidences of self-transcendence. Bloomfield (1980) has suggested that spiritual health and well being are best described as "an overall sense of personal fulfillment and satisfaction with life, a sense of peace with oneself and the world . . . a sense of unity with the cosmos or of personal closeness to God, or with nature" (p. 25).

Welwood (1986b) has delineated mature personality characteristics that are indicative of a spiritually healthy person. They are compassion, discernment, generosity, patience, and wisdom (p. 288). In describing spiritual health in terms of vital aliveness, access to life-force energy, and the achievement of high levels of moral development, including a capacity for inclusiveness and principled living (Cowley, 1996a), the trend toward seeming spiritual maturation as a developmental achievement continued.

WILBER'S FULL SPECTRUM OF CONSCIOUSNESS MODEL

With his first book, Ken Wilber challenged Western concepts of optimum human potential (that culminated with the development of a strong ego) by positing what he called "a full spectrum of consciousness" (Wilber, 1977). Over the years, Wilber has continued to refine his ideas about the developmental possibilities inherent in the human species by proposing a spectrum psychology or unified theory of development (Wilber, 1999). By understanding the level of development of a client, the therapist can be much more effective in choosing appropriate interventions (Cowley, 1996a). For this reason, Wilber's Full Spectrum of Consciousness Model, as proposed in 1986, is an especially helpful one for clinical practitioners. It integrated psychological and developmental theories of the East and the West across three general levels of consciousness (prepersonal, personal, and transpersonal). It also proposed a view of which pathologies might occur at each developmental level. Wilber even suggested which interventions might work best for clinical work with developmental problems at each of the three levels of consciousness:

> Psychotherapy, as I see it, is applied developmental psychology. The therapist uses his or her knowledge of normal development to reach some conclusions about the reasons for a patient's malfunctioning and how one may enter the developmental spiral either to foster or to reinsti-

tute a more productive, or at least less destructive, developmental process. (Basch, 1988, p. 29)

Since a strong grounding in developmental theory helps one pinpoint more accurately the client's level of consciousness or functioning, it behooves us to take a closer look at Wilber's Full Spectrum of Consciousness Model.

The three general levels of Wilber's 1986 Model (prepersonal, personal, and transpersonal) roughly correspond to Freud's three levels of the psyche: *it* (id), *I* (ego), and *Above I* (superego) (Bettelheim, 1983). Assagioli, a contemporary of Freud, also designated three levels of consciousness that he labeled lower consciousness, middle consciousness, and superconsciousness that (1965). By further exploring Wilber's three levels of consciousness, it is apparent how compatible they are with earlier models.

The prepersonal level of consciousness is an undeveloped level wherein the person has no firm sense of personal identity. In such a fluid self-system, self and object representations tend to merge or fuse (Wilber, 1986). This primitive level of development is characterized by prerational structures, impulses, and primary processes commonly associated with early childhood development. After approximately age three, if the above descriptors apply to a person's level of functioning, then the existence of psychotic, narcissistic, borderline personality disorders, and/or psychoneurotic ego structures may be indicated.

The personal level of consciousness is characterized by a beginning sense of rational-individuated-personal selfhood wherein the individual experiences a sense of identity and relative autonomy. This level includes, at the upper limits, a well-developed value structure of a self-actualized person.

The transpersonal level of consciousness includes those stages of human development that go beyond ego and self-actualization toward self-transcendence. This stage is characterized by consistently mature (if not saint-like) character traits like generativity, altruism, compassion, and the capacity for unconditional love.

Vaughan (1987) has also identified descriptors of different levels of development along the spectrum of consciousness. In her view, ego transcendence (or the transpersonal level of consciousness) is characterized by: (a) integrated, articulated wholeness in contrast to undifferentiated oneness; (b) consciously cognized intuition in contrast to trance or passive, unconscious perception; (c) faith and grace in contrast to infantile dependence; (d) insight in contrast to undifferentiated perception; (e) spontaneity in contrast to reactivity and impulsiveness; (f) altruism in contrast to narcissism; and (g) purity of heart in contrast to ignorance (p. 270).

By developing criteria that delineate between levels of development and functioning along the spectrum of consciousness, transpersonal theorists are providing some useful guidelines for practitioners about how to differentiate between optimally healthy experiences that go beyond ego (path), and processes that are unhealthy, repressive, or blatantly psychotic (pathology).

A Continuum of Psychopathology

Even though most traditional theorists tend to contain their accounts of serious pathology to the prepersonal levels, Wilber (1986) has pointed out that "this by no means exhausts the spectrum of pathologies, not even the spectrum of 'serious' or 'profound' pathologies" (p. 114). The Full Spectrum of Consciousness Model not only extended psychological understanding of human potential beyond ego and self-actualization toward self-transcendence, it also expanded understanding of what psychopathology may look like at personal/existential and transpersonal levels of consciousness.

Personal Level Psychopathology. Some of the pathologies associated with the personal level of Wilber's developmental model include role conflict and script neurosis. In role conflict, the use of duplicitous transactions (overtly communicating one message while covertly implying another) and/or hidden agendas, emerge as prime defense mechanisms. Wilber (1986) warns that if these modes of coping are extreme, they may result in "an interior splitting, or dissociation" of the self (p. 115). Identity neuroses are also potentially regressive or pathological trends identified at the personal level. As cognitive structures become more abstract and complex, and self-development becomes more differentiated, the emerging self may be overcome with anxiety or depression. Philosophical questions and challenges can wear down one's ego structure, leaving the person crippled with doubt:

> "Identity neurosis" specifically means all of the things that can go wrong in the emergence of this self-reflective structure. Is it strong enough to break free of the rule/role mind and stand on its own principles of conscience? Can it, if necessary, summon the courage to march to the sound of a different drummer? Will it dare to think for itself? Will it be overcome with anxiety or depression at the prospect of its own emergence? (Wilber, 1986, p. 116)

At the upper limits of the personal level, existential pathologies may emerge. For example, Frankl (1968, 1975), Fabry (1980), and Krill (1996) have provided excellent descriptions of existential pathologies wherein a sense of alienation, meaninglessness, and/or inauthenticity can plunge a person into existential despair and inhibit healthy functioning.

Transpersonal Level Psychopathology. It is in the delineation and description of pathologies of the spiritual or transpersonal realm that Wilber has broken new ground and provided clinicians with important understandings requisite to practice with the spiritual dimension. His Full Spectrum of Consciousness Model (1986) posited three hierarchical sub-levels within the transpersonal domain, which he referred to as psychic, subtle, and causal. Sometimes Wilber includes the "ultimate" or "non-dual" as a fourth level within the transpersonal domain. This article deals only with the three levels posited in Wilber's 1986 model since "strictly speaking, the ultimate is not one level among others, but the reality, condition, or suchness of all levels" (Wilber, 1999, p. 88).

Transpersonal pathologies may occur at each of the three sub-levels within the transpersonal dimension. Wilber (1986) posited that each sub-level exhibits different kinds of spiritual pathology with clearly discernable symptoms that require differential remedies (p. 145). He emphasized that his ideas about transpersonal pathology are offered as the result of "a preliminary investigation." He further points out that he does this "not as a series of dogmatic conclusions but as a way to open the discussion on a topic that has been sorely neglected by conventional and contemplative schools alike" (p. 119).

At the lowest transpersonal sub-level of consciousness (psychic), spiritual crises and pathologies may emerge spontaneously with "extremely unbalancing results" (p. 120) for individuals who have just begun their journey up the ladder of being. Dramatic psychosomatic symptoms may include muscle spasms, violent headaches, and difficulty breathing. Psychologically, pathology at the psychic level may be expressed as free-floating anxiety, egoitis (psychic inflation), a dark night of the soul (psychic depression), or pranic disorders associated with the spontaneous rising of kundalini energies and/or the practice of a spiritual discipline like yoga. "The great intensity of psychic and subtle energies, can, as it were, overload the 'lower circuits' resulting in everything from allergies to intestinal problems, to heart disorders" (Wilber, 1986, p. 122).

Pathology at the subtle sub-level of transpersonal consciousness results from an inability to let go of the mental-psychic self in order to identify and integrate with Divine Presence or one's own archetype/essential nature (Wilber, 1986). According to Wilber, this failure to transform represents a kind of "fixation" or "morbid preservation." Morbid preservation occurs when the once appropriate identifications and object relations of a particular level are not released to allow room for newer and higher ones. Whenever one makes an exclusive identification with a particular level of consciousness, one's evolutionary progress toward realization of the higher Self is put on hold leaving the person "stranded on the shores of its own agony" (p. 124).

Causal sub-level transpersonal disorders include failure of differentiation from ego. When one is unable to accept the final death of the separate self, the result is a failure to integrate the manifest and unmanifest realms. Since so few people have ever achieved the causal level of transpersonal development, treating its pathologies is not likely to become a common problem for practitioners. Whenever pathologies of the transpersonal level are identified, a referral to a practitioner knowledgeable about transpersonal interventions is recommended.

Three Levels of Interventions

Since the pathologies of each level (and sub-level) of consciousness are stage-specific, interventions must be chosen with careful discrimination:

> It is important to emphasize again the great care that should ideally be given to differential diagnosis, particularly in light of the full spectrum of human growth and development. For example, psychic anxiety, existential anxiety, psychoneurotic anxiety, and borderline anxiety are apparently very different phenomena with very different treatment modalities, and thus any effective and appropriate therapeutic intervention depends significantly on an accurate initial diagnosis. This, in turn, rests upon a skilled understanding of the overall levels of self-structuralization and the particular types of needs, motivations, cognitions, object relations, defense mechanisms, and pathologies that are specific and characteristic for each stage of structural development and organization. (Wilber, 1986, p.146)

To get an in-depth understanding of Wilber's model, one needs to study his original works. For the purposes of this article, a brief summation of three general levels of intervention will be presented. (For more detail, see Wilber, 1986, p. 145; Cowley, 1996a, pp. 692-693.)

1. *Interventions at the prepersonal level* range from medication or pacification for psychotic disorders to ego structure building for narcissistic-borderline disorders.

> It is often said that the aim of therapy in these less-than-neurotically structured clients is to enable them to reach the level of neurosis, repression, and resistance. . . . The aim of the structure-building techniques, very simply, is to help the individual re-engage and complete the separation-individuation process. (Wilber, 1986, p. 128)

Once a person has achieved enough ego structure to repress, some "uncovering" techniques may be utilized at the psychoneurotic level. Since much of the work at this prepersonal level of development is psychodynamic in nature,

First Force therapies (e.g., psychoanalytic, self or ego psychology, object relations, etc.) are usually the treatments of choice.

2. *Interventions at the personal level* are usually drawn from Second Force (behavioral and cognitive behavioral theories) and Third Force (humanistic, experiential, and existential) theories. Problems at the personal level, such as role confusion, cognitive distortions, and role/rule pathologies, respond well to interventions from transactional analysis and cognitive behavioral therapies. At the upper limits of the personal level, existential depression, angst, inauthenticity, ennui, and the like are ameliorated with person-centered interventions like gestalt and creative visualization. Existential interventions, such as Socratic dialogue and logotherapy (among others), can be utilized to help client systems make meaning of their lives and become more autonomous as they move toward actualization of their highest potential.

3. *Interventions at the transpersonal level* include methods used to strengthen and purify the body-mind-spirit. They may include exercise, maintaining a special diet, meditation, and/or pursuit of contemplative practice with a spiritual teacher.

Hindrances to Spiritual Practice

When working with the spiritual dimension, it is important not only to understand what pathologies might occur and how to intervene based on the level of consciousness involved, but also to understand obstacles to spiritual maturation that client systems may encounter. Grof and Grof (1989) have discussed some of the common obstacles, vicissitudes, and hindrances that may thwart spiritual evolution:

> For it often happens that people, in their spiritual practice or in the course of everyday life, encounter phases of their inner development in which things fall apart. . . . Of course these "crises" are experienced not just by people undertaking systematic spiritual practice, but also by many persons who in the course of their lives have a natural spiritual awakening. They can be brought on by many things, such as death of an important person, childbirth, a powerful sexual experience, or having a near-death accident and realizing through an out-of-body experience that you are not this physical body. At other times, they can be triggered by the illuminations that come through spending time in the high mountains or through a difficult divorce or some life-threatening illness like cancer. (p. 140)

Just as it was written that demonic hosts tried to prevent The Buddha's quest for enlightenment, so it also seems that life itself sometimes conspires to place hindrances or difficult states of mind in one's path to sabotage self-transcendence. How can therapists help their clients to recognize some of the stumbling blocks along the spiritual path?

> In order to work with our hindrances we must identify them clearly. The first is *desire* and *wanting*. The second is its opposite, which is *aversion*–anger and dislike, judgment and fear–all those states that push away experience. The next pair is *sleepiness, dullness,* and *lethargy,* or resistance to experience, and their opposite, which is *agitation* and restlessness of mind. The fifth is *doubt,* the part of the mind that says, "I cannot do it. It is too hard. . . . " (Grof & Grof, 1989, p. 143)

According to the Grofs, working to overcome hindrances to spiritual development is basically a matter of becoming skilled observers and not allowing the self to identify with any particular mental or emotional state because it is recognized as being impermanent and transitory. Rising above hindrances requires an intentional shift of consciousness to higher or more mature ways of thinking and behaving. The Grofs (1989) identified five specific antidotes influenced by Buddhist teachings that can be utilized in working with obstacles to spiritual development:

1. "Let be."
2. Sublimate or transform the difficult energy outwardly or inwardly.
3. Appropriately use suppression until a proper circumstance arises for you to deal directly with the issue.
4. Explore the difficulties through the tactics of imagination and exaggeration to see what they may have to teach you.
5. Pay attention, and act out of the mind state with awareness and mindfulness. (pp. 147-148)

Spirituality and the DSM IV

In 1994, the American Psychiatric Association added a V code (V62.895) relative to religious and spiritual problems. Including this category among conditions meriting treatment–but distinguishing them from mental disorders–served notice that although the spiritual domain is a legitimate dimension to be included in making a multidimensional assessment, difficulties related to religion and spirituality may be normal problems of living, as opposed to inherently pathological conditions. Thus work with religious and spiritual issues requires the practitioner to make distinctions between spiritually healthy manifestations within normal development and distortions or pathologies that may appear in the process of spiritual development.

It may be tempting to discount unfamiliar concepts from Wilber's transpersonal theory as not having relevance for our profession or the client systems that we serve. Since transpersonal theory integrates psychologies of both the East and the West, some of the words and concepts will inevitably sound foreign and strange to us. However, Vaughan (1987) reminded us: "While we are working on expanding our perceptual framework, it behooves us to be aware of the limitations of our ability to pass judgment on teachers and teachings we have not been trained to evaluate" (p. 277).

Transpersonal psychology is beginning to acquire a transdisciplinary nature (Nalimov & Drogalina, 1996). It not only challenges us to expand our vocabulary but also to make some shifts in conceptual frameworks. This is what Arrien predicted in 1993 would be our work as we go into the 21st century–"a time of bridging ancient wisdoms into the creative tapestry of contemporary times" (p. 11).

The expansion of social work practice to redefine the relationship between spirituality and mental illness or health will require the incorporation into social work education of various theories and models that include the spiritual dimension. Additionally, more case study research is required to ascertain and document the effectiveness of Fourth Force clinical interventions (Cowley, 1996a). If, as Wilber (1999) has suggested, it takes decades and maybe centuries (p. 178) to incorporate a new paradigm, we have our work cut out for us.

REFERENCES

Anthony, D., Ecker, B., & Wilber, L. (Eds.). (1987). *Spiritual choices: The problem of recognizing authentic paths to inner transformation.* New York: Paragon House Publishers.

Arrien, A. (1993). *The four-fold way.* San Francisco: Harper.

Assagioli, R. (1965). *Psychosynthesis.* New York: Viking Press.

Basch, M. (1988). *Understanding psychotherapy: The science behind the art.* New York: Basic Books.

Bettelheim, B. (1983). *Freud and man's soul.* New York: Alfred A. Knopf.

Bloomfield, H. (1980). Transcendental meditation as an adjunct to therapy. In S. Boorstein (Ed.), *Transpersonal psychology* (pp. 123-140). Palo Alto, CA: Science and Behavior Books.

Boorstein, S. (1996). *Transpersonal techniques and psychology.* New York: Basic Books.

Brothers, B. (1992). *Spirituality and couples: Heart and soul in the therapeutic process.* New York: The Haworth Press, Inc.

Bucke, R. (1923). *Cosmic consciousness: A study of the evolution of the human mind.* New York: D. P. Dutton.

Bullis, R. (1996). *Spirituality in social work practice.* Washington, DC: Taylor & Francis.

Campbell, J. (Ed.). (1971). *The portable Jung.* New York: Viking Press.

Canda, E. (1988a). Conceptualizing spirituality for social work: Insights from diverse perspectives. *Social Thought, 13*(1), 30-46.

Canda, E. (1988b). Spirituality, religious diversity, and social work practice. *Social Casework, 69*(4), 238-247.

Canda, E. (1989). Religious content in social work education: A comparative approach. *Journal of Social Work Education, 25*(1), 36-45.

Canda, E., & Chambers, D. (1994). Should spiritual principles guide social policy? Yes. In H. Karger & J. Midgley (Eds.), *Controversial issues in social policy* (pp. 63-70, 74-78). Boston: Allyn & Bacon.

Canda, E., & Furman, L. (1999). *Spiritual diversity in social work practice: The heart of helping.* New York: The Free Press.

Cowley, A. (1993). Transpersonal social work: A theory for the 1990s. *Social Work, 28*(5), 527-534.

Cowley, A. (1996a). Transpersonal practice: A fourth force model. In F. Turner (Ed.), *Social work treatment: Interlocking theoretical approaches* (4th ed., pp. 663-698). New York: The Free Press.

Cowley, A. (1996b). Expressing the soul of social work. *Society for Spirituality and Social Work Newsletter, 3*(2), 1, 6-8.

Cowley, A. (1999). Transpersonal theory and social work practice with couples and families. *Journal of Family Social Work, 2*(2), 5-21.

Cowley, A., & Derezotes, D. (1994). Transpersonal psychology and social work education. *Journal of Social Work Education, 30*(4), 32-41.

Derezotes, D. (2000). *Advanced generalist social work practice.* Thousand Oaks, CA: Sage.

Fabry, J. (1980). Use of the transpersonal in logotherapy. In S. Boorstein (Ed.), *Transpersonal psychology.* Palo Alto, CA: Science & Behavior Books.

Frankl, V. (1968). *The doctor and the soul.* New York: Knopf.

Frankl, V. (1975). *The unconscious god.* New York: Simon & Schuster.

Freud, S. (1946). *Totem and taboo.* New York: Vintage.

Grof, S., & Grof, C. (1989). *Spiritual emergency: When personal transformation becomes a crisis.* Los Angeles: Jeremy P. Tarcher, Inc.

Hendlin, S. (1985). The spiritual emergency patient: Concept and example. In E.M. Stem (Ed.), *Transpersonal approaches to counseling and psychotherapy.* Denver: Love Publishing.

James, W. (1961). The *varieties of religious experience.* New York: Colliers.

Joseph, V. (1987). The religious and spiritual aspects of clinical practice: A neglected dimension of social work. *Social Thought, 13*(1), 12-23.

Krill, D. (1996). Existential social work. In F. Turner (Ed.), *Social work treatment: Interlocking theoretical approaches* (4th ed., pp. 250-281). New York: The Free Press.

Liester, M. (1996). Inner voices distinguishing transcendent and pathological characteristics. *The Journal of Transpersonal Psychology, 28*(1), 1-30.

London, P. (1986). *The modes and morals of psychotherapy.* New York: Hemisphere Publishing Corporation.

Lukoff, D., Lu, F., & Turner, R. (1996). Diagnosis: A transpersonal clinical approach to religious and spiritual problems. In B. Scotton, A. Chinen, & J. Batista (Eds.), *Textbook of transpersonal psychiatry and psychology.* New York: Basic Books.

Marx, K. (1906). *Das Kapital: Resemblances between the psychic lives of savages and neurotics.* Chicago: C.H. Carr & Company.

Nalimov, V., & Drogalina, J. (1996). The transpersonal movement: A Russian perspective on its emergence and prospects for further development. *The Journal of Transpersonal Psychology, 28*(1), 49-62.

Peay, P. (1997). The world at the door. *Common Boundary, 32-39.*

Peck, M. S. (1978). *The road less traveled.* New York: Simon & Schuster.

Robbins, S., Chatterjee, P., & Canda, E. (1998). *Contemporary human behavior theory.* Boston: Allyn & Bacon.

Russel, R. (1998). Spirituality and religion in graduate social work education. In E. Canda (Ed.), *Spirituality in social work: New directions.* New York: The Haworth Press, Inc.

Sheridan, M., Bullis, R., Adcock, C., Berlin, S., & Miller, P. (1992). Practitioners' personal and professional attitudes toward religion and spirituality: Issues for education and practice. *Journal of Social Work Education, 28*(2),190-203.

Swedenborg, E. (1872). *Heaven and its wonders, the world of spirits and hell: From things heard and seen.* New York: American Swendenborg Printing and Publishing Society.

Vaughan, F. (1987). A question of balance: Health and pathology in new religious movements. In Anthony et al. (Eds.), *Spiritual choices: The problem of recognizing authentic paths to inner transformation.* New York: Paragon House.

Vaughan, F. (1995). Spiritual freedom. *The Quest, 8*(4), 48-55.

Wade, J. (1996). *Changes of Mind: A holonomic theory of the evolution of consciousness.* New York: State University of New York Press.

Walsh, R., & Vaughan, F. (1980). *Beyond ego: Transpersonal dimensions in psychology.* Los Angeles: Jeremy P. Tarcher, Inc.

Walsh, R., & Vaughan, F. (1993). The art of transcendence: An introduction to common elements of transpersonal practice. *The Journal of Transpersonal Psychology, 25*(1), 1-9.

West, D. (1985). *Cosmic Consciousness.* (Unpublished paper, Graduate School of Social Work, University of Utah at Salt Lake City).

Wilber, K. (1977). *The spectrum of consciousness.* Wheaton, IL: Quest Publications.

Wilber, K. (1980). The pre/trans fallacy. *ReVision, 3,* 51-73.

Wilber, K. (1986). The spectrum of development, the spectrum of psychopathology, & treatment modalities. In K. Wilber, J. Engler, & D. Brown (Eds.), *Transformations of consciousness* (pp. 65-159). Boston: New Science Library/Shambhala.

Wilber, K. (1999). *The collected works of Ken Wilber* (Vol. 4). Boston & London: Shambhala.

The Relationship Between Spiritual Development and Ethnicity in Violent Men

Dexter R. Freeman

SUMMARY. There is a dearth of empirically based literature on spirituality and how it impacts the behavior of violent men. In fact, domestic violence practitioners and researchers often diminish the influence of spirituality in the lives of violent men and assume that violent men, regardless of their ethnicity, can be accurately understood using Eurocentric paradigms that de-emphasize the importance of spirituality. This article reveals that the lack of attention that has been given to spirituality may be negating a significant resource for violent men, especially among African American men. It provides empirical data on the spiritual perspectives of African American and European American men. It also shows that the spiritual energies that promote a sense of wholeness have a significant influence on the level of physical violence used by violent men, regardless of their ethnic identity. *[Article copies available for a fee from The Haworth Document Delivery Service: 1-800-342-9678. E-mail address: <getinfo@haworthpressinc.com> Website: <http://www.HaworthPress.com> © 2001 by The Haworth Press, Inc. All rights reserved.]*

KEYWORDS. Spirituality, archetypal, violence, transpersonal, ethnicity, social work

Dexter R. Freeman, PhD, LCSW, is Chief of the Soldier and Family Support Branch at the Army Medical Department Center and School, MCCS-HPS, 3151 Scott Road, Fort Sam Houston, TX 78234 (E-mail: dexfree@earthlink.net or dexter.freeman@amedd.army.mil).

[Haworth co-indexing entry note]: "The Relationship Between Spiritual Development and Ethnicity in Violent Men." Freeman, Dexter R. Co-published simultaneously in *Social Thought* (The Haworth Press, Inc.) Vol. 20, No. 1/2, 2001, pp. 95-107; and: *Transpersonal Perspectives on Spirituality in Social Work* (ed: Edward R. Canda, and Elizabeth D. Smith) The Haworth Press Inc., 2001, pp. 95-107. Single or multiple copies of this article are available for a fee from The Haworth Document Delivery Service [1-800-342-9678, 9:00 a.m. - 5:00 p.m. (EST). E-mail address: getinfo@haworthpressinc.com].

INTRODUCTION

Although a large percentage of domestic violence clients are African American, most theories and research on domestic violence are derived from Eurocentric paradigms (Clark, Beckett, Wells, & Dungee-Anderson, 1994; Forte, Franks, Forte, & Rigsby, 1996). These theories, unlike the African worldview, de-emphasize the importance of spirituality and elevate the significance of rugged individualism, competitiveness, power and control, and intellectualism. Moreover, they view violence as linear in its origination (Warfield-Coppock, 1995). This article considers whether practitioners who ascribe to theories and practice models that exclude spirituality can truly understand the worldview of African American men who have been violent.

Some writers contend that African Americans are ostensibly Westernized Africans who have incorporated the Eurocentric worldview (Swigonski, 1996). Therefore, they believe that African American and European American violent men can be effectively understood and assisted using similar paradigms. Other writers believe that African Americans have retained their Afrocentric perspective that emphasizes spirituality, connectedness, and a belief that true harmony occurs only by maintaining a balance with others and the divine (Asante, 1988; Vanzant, 1996). The African worldview is a holistic perspective that includes a oneness of mind, body, and spirit; a collective rather than individual identity; and a perception that the cause for phenomena, such as violence, must be viewed as annular or circular rather than linear (Kamya, 1997; Swigonski, 1996).

This article addresses two questions: Is there a difference between the spiritual perspectives of African American and European American violent men? Also, does spiritual development effect the level of physical violence used by violent men across ethnic groups?

Spirituality

Spirituality, although often neglected by mental health practitioners, is central to human existence (Hammerschlag, 1993; Washburn, 1995). It is a primary ingredient that serves to make people unique and connected at the same time. Joseph (1987) referred to spirituality as the underlying dimension of consciousness that strives for meaning, union with the universe, and with all things. Vaughan (1991) described spirituality as the genesis of compassion, gratitude, awareness of a transcendent dimension, and an appreciation for life which brings meaning and purpose.

Spiritual development encompasses a universal search for a state of wholeness or completeness that includes a conglomeration of masculine and feminine energies, strengths and weaknesses, and internal and external forces that operate to serve a divine purpose. Wholeness dictates an integration of transpersonal energies that compel people to seek an understanding of their true meaning and a connection with the sacred and divine. Jung (1959) believed the degree which one develops spiritually to experience wholeness is contingent upon one's awareness of the spiritual energies or archetypes that are within the collective unconscious, which is synonymous with the soul and spirit. However, when one fails to embrace spiritual (archetypal) energies within the collective unconscious, these forces begin influencing one's perspective in a negative manner. Therefore, spiritual energies are not only constructive, but can also be destructive, shadowy forces, if they are rejected (Singer, 1994).

Jung (1959) described the collective unconscious as a non-personal aggregate of spiritual energies (archetypes) that are innate and universal. This non-personal energy governs one's perspective and view of the world (Hillman, 1975). The collective unconscious contains archetypes, which are numinous, transformative, and powerful primordial images that are not observed directly, but are recognized by their effect (Smith, 1990). No archetype is better than another, and each one is integral to the experience of wholeness.

Spiritual Development

Washburn's (1995) dynamic-dialectical transpersonal theory and Pearson's (1991) heroic myth archetypal theory described a triphasic quest for wholeness or spiritual development that is universal. Pearson (1991) stated that these levels of spiritual development occur at the ego, soul, and self or spirit levels. Pearson (1991) and Washburn (1995) also elucidated how archetypes or spiritual energies are available throughout the triphasic journey. They explained that even though archetypal energy is non-personal, in that it is everywhere and originates from the dynamic (spiritual) ground or collective unconscious, it must be incorporated into an individual's state of consciousness in order for one to develop a greater sense of wholeness.

Washburn (1995) postulated that we are all spiritual beings at birth–deeply embedded with the spiritual ground from which we were created. Pearson (1991) referred to the period of development when individuals innately seek to discover a sense of security within themselves and their environment as the ego level of spiritual development. It is important to recognize that an unquantifiable amount of archetypal energy is available at the ego development level. These energies engender multiple perspectives that result in a healthy ego. Pearson (1991) identified four ego level archetypes (Innocent, Orphan, Warrior, and Caregiver) which promote child-like and primary adult-like perspectives that are paramount to developing an ego that is healthy enough to endure the journey into the soul and spirit levels of development.

Table 1 outlines these ego-level archetypes, their purpose, and the gifts or perspectives they provide. The Innocent and Orphan archetypes emit child-like spiritual energies that enable one to experience security based upon a balance between the acknowledgment of faith or trust and the acceptance of reality (Pearson, 1991). The Warrior and Caregiver are primary adult-like spiritual energies that enable one to recognize responsibilities toward oneself and others by appropriately confronting challenges and nurturing oneself and others when the need arises (Pearson, 1991).

When a crisis occurs, or a significant loss is experienced, an individual will tend to question oneself and one's perspective of the world. These thoughts are indicative of messages from spiritual energy at the soul level. Hillman (1992) explained that the soul searches for meaning in the midst of pain and destruction. It connects one with the eternal and provides a sense of meaning and value to life. Archetypal energy at the soul level provides enlightenment so that one might understand what is most important. It helps one respond authentically. This energy also compels people to seek their true loves and passions in life, thereby embracing destruction (i.e., letting go of identifying with prior beliefs, values, and images) which is tantamount to celebrating the life that they were meant to have (Pearson, 1991; Roberts, 1992).

While the second level of spiritual development (growth at the soul level) promotes an awareness of one's true meaning and purpose in life, level three (growth at the spirit level) brings freedom and power that results from experiencing wholeness. However, the spirit level cannot be experienced in a healthy manner by everyone. Many people are hampered in experiencing this level of spiritual development due to the presence of shadows (i.e., spiritual energy

TABLE 1. Ego-level Archetypes: Gifts and Goals

Archetype	Goal	Fear	Gift
Innocent	remain safe	abandonment	trust, hope, loyalty, commitment
Orphan	regain safety	exploitation	realism, independence, vulnerability
Warrior	win	weakness	courage, discipline, challenge
Caregiver	help others	selfishness	compassion, nurture, generosity

Note. The source for this information is Pearson, C. (1991).

that is repressed or denied and influences one's perspective negatively) and unresolved issues at the ego and soul levels.

Spiritual energy at the spirit level provides a perspective that helps people experience freedom and power through achieving a sense of oneness with God, the universe, community, or the cosmos (Pearson, 1991). The principal features of this stage are: (a) experiencing transcendence and an integration of major dualisms that may have plagued the ego, i.e., the masculine versus feminine, logic versus emotionalism, and dependence versus independence; (b) having a spiritual presence or charisma; and (c) an agapic sense of oneness within and with the environment, cosmos, or the divine (Pearson, 1991; Washburn, 1995).

Ethnicity and Spiritual Development

African Americans tend to be spirit focused and their humanity is usually viewed collectively, rather than individually (Carter, 1999; Daly, Jennings, Beckett, & Leashore, 1995). Furthermore, ethnographers often identify spirituality as a key factor for coping with stress among African Americans (Haight, 1998). Therefore, African American men have a strong proclivity towards viewing themselves and their experiences according to their connection with others and the communal consciousness (Rasheed & Rasheed, 1999). Moreover, the recognition of God or a divine being is valued and central to the existence of most African Americans. Traditionally, African Americans view God as omnipotent, benevolent, and a source of miraculous power–capable of rectifying pain, sorrow, and injustice (Reese, Ahern, Nair, O'Faire, & Warren, 1999). In addition, Pearson (1991) postulated that African cultures tend to be opened to the soul and spirit level energies more than European cultures.

The Afrocentric worldview values interrelatedness, connectedness, and interdependence; faith in a transcendental force; an acceptance of oneself and other members of the community; and the belief that there is a natural order or underlying principle that governs the cosmos (Kamya, 1997; Swigonski, 1996). However, the Eurocentric world values competitiveness, materialism, value boundaries, and human control of the world (Warfield-Coppock, 1995). It is also ego oriented, assuming that few things are more important than an understanding of oneself.

METHODOLOGY

Hypotheses and Design

This cross-sectional study utilized analysis of variance (ANOVA) to determine if there was a difference between the spiritual perspectives of African

American men and European American men. Bivariate correlation analyses were also performed to determine if ethnicity and the components of spiritual development were related to the level of physical violence used by violent men.

The study hypothesized that controlling for age, alcoholism, income level, and time in treatment, there would be a significant difference between the spiritual perspectives of African Americans and European Americans. European Americans would be more identified with the spiritual (archetypal) energy at the ego level than African Americans. However, African Americans would be more aware of spiritual energy at the soul and spirit levels than European Americans. Therefore, African Americans would be less aware of the Innocent, Orphan, Warrior, and Caregiver archetypal energies than European Americans. However, African Americans would be more aware of spiritual energy that promotes an awareness of one's purpose or meaning in life and spiritual energy that enables one to connect with the divine (God).

Sample

Self-report questionnaires were completed anonymously by 133 men who were in treatment for domestic violence in Northern Virginia and Central Maryland. The participants had a mean age of 33.4 and ranged from 19 to 60. The majority of the men (61%) were European American, and 23% of the participants were African American. Other ethnic groups (16%) included a small number of Indigenous (Native) Americans, Asian Americans, Hispanic Americans, and those with mixed heritage. Forty-three percent of the men identified themselves as Protestant, 27% were affiliated with the Catholic faith, and 15% held no religious affiliation. On average, the participants were well educated, with 44% having education beyond high school. In addition, the majority (72%) of the participants were court mandated into treatment.

Study Measures

Heroic Myth Index (Modified). A modified version of Pearson's (1991) Heroic Myth Index (HMI) was used to measure the extent the participants were aware of archetypes at the ego level of spiritual development. The HMI scales measured how active the Innocent, Orphan, Warrior, and Caregiver archetypes (see Table 1) were in the lives of the participants. Each archetypal scale was scored separately, with a possible score that ranged from 5 to 25. Low scores (from 5 to 13) were suggestive of an archetype that was active in an individual's life as a shadow. Thus when an individual experiences this archetype it tends to affect him or her in a negative manner. A mid-range score (14 to 19) indicated that an individual was ambivalent or indifferent about identifying with that archetype. A high score (20 to 25) revealed an archetype that was consciously active in an individual's life. Cronbach's Alpha Test revealed that all the HMI scales were reliable above .50, thus making them acceptable for research purposes (Caplan, Naidu & Tripathi, 1984). The Innocent was reliable at .56, Orphan at .82, Warrior at .63, and Caregiver at .74.

Existential Well-Being Scale. Growth at the soul level was measured using Ellison's (1983) Existential Well-Being Scale (EWBS). Hillman (1972) defined the soul as an unconscious force that makes meaning possible, turns events into experiences, and is communicated in love. The soul connects people with the eternal and provides a sense of meaning and value to life (Pearson, 1991). The EWBS is a 10 item scale, with a possible score range from 10 to 60. This scale has been effective in identifying the degree to which people perceive their life has purpose and meaning (Crandall & Rasmussen, 1975; Ellison, 1983). The reliability of the EWBS was .84 in this study.

Religious Well-Being Scale. Growth at the spirit level was measured using Ellison's (1983) Religious Well-Being Scale (RWBS). Washburn (1995) described the spirit level as the phase that enables people to experience a state of oneness within and a connection with God. The RWBS is a 10 item scale, with a possible score range from 10 to 60, that measures the level of connection or relationship one has with God. The higher the participants scored on the RWBS, the stronger their relationship with God. The RWBS had a reliability of .89.

Physical Violence Scale (PVS). The PVS, from the Conflict Tactic Scales, is one of the most reliable and effective instruments for measuring family violence (Straus & Gelles, 1990). The PVS, a 9 item scale with a possible scoring range from 0 to 54, was used to assess the participants' use of physical violence. The higher a participant scored, the greater the level of physical violence they used within the past 12 months. The Physical Violence Scale (PVS) had a reliability coefficient of .90.

Control Variables

The control variables, age, income level, and time in treatment, were assessed using standard demographic questions on the research questionnaire. Alcoholism was assessed using the Short Michigan Alcoholism Screening Test (SMAST). The SMAST is a 13 item questionnaire that measures the level of alcoholism (Magruder-Habid, Durand, & Frey, 1991). A score of 5 or greater suggests alcoholism. The SMAST had a reliability of .78 in this study.

FINDINGS

Prior studies have shown that as people age, they tend to have fewer ego concerns, be more comfortable with themselves, and express a greater sense of meaning and purpose. Also, as men and women age, they tend to experience more balance in their personalities, and men tend to use less violence (Grove, Ortega, & Style, 1989; O'Leary, 1999). Similarly, bivariate correlation analysis in this study showed that younger participants were more violent than older participants (see Table 2). Alcohol abuse was also significantly related to the use of physical violence among the participants in this study. The more the participants had problems that were alcohol related, the more likely they were to use physical violence.

In addition, Table 2 also shows that there was a significant linear relationship between the participants' use of physical violence and their identification with spiritual energies at the ego and soul (EWBS) levels of spiritual development. The more the participants embraced the spiritual energies that promoted their sense of purpose, the less physical violence they used. Also, the more the participants embraced Caregiver energy (the spiritual energy that promotes a perspective that encourages people to nurture themselves and others), the less physical violence they used. However, the more the participants became aware of Orphan energy (the spiritual energy that promotes a perspective that enables one to feel separate, independent, helpless, and vulnerable), the more physical violence the participants used.

TABLE 2. Correlations Between Variables and Physical Violence

Variables	Afro-American	Euro-American	Total Pop.
Age	−.11	−.19	−.19*
Income	.02	.02	−.08
Alcohol	.13	.22	.23**
Time	.22	−.14	−.09
Innocent	−.21	.18	−.07
Orphan	.04	.35**	.30**
Caregiver	−.29	−.29**	−.23**
Warrior	.33	−.05	−.12
EWBS	−.31	−.26*	−.26**
RWBS	−.34	−.10	.003

Note. The total population consists of African Americans, European Americans, and other minorities.
*indicates p < .05 and **indicates p < .01.

Table 3 reveals the mean scores for ego level spiritual energies. These results show that the participants were ambivalent towards embracing Innocent, Warrior, and Caregiver energy. These results are consistent with other studies that identified violent men as fearful of abandonment, non-assertive, distrusting, holding idealistic views towards the world, and having difficulties asking for and exhibiting affection (Dutton, 1995; Paymar, 1993).

The participants' mean scores on the Orphan scale were indicative of a shadow archetype. As such, the participants would tend to use negative or self-destructive behavior to distance themselves from this energy when it surfaces. The bivariate correlation analysis (see Table 2) supports the finding that the low score on the Orphan scale is reflective of an archetype that controls the participants as a shadow. These findings highlight the importance of violent men acknowledging in a constructive way the weak and vulnerable spiritual energy (Orphan) that they often try to avoid.

TABLE 3. Comparison of Means by Ethnic Groups

Variables	Total Pop.	African	European	Other	Sig.
Age	33.3	33.7	33.4	32.5	.875
Income	2.2	1.9	2.3	2.1	.275
Alcohol	7.9	8.5	8.0	6.8	.752
Time	1.2	1.4	1.2	1.1	.55
Innocent	14.4	14.3	14.2	15.5	.261
Orphan	12.2	11.8	12.1	13.1	.615
Warrior	17.9	17.1	18.1	18.2	.443
Caregiver	18.1	18.3	17.8	19.0	.386
EWBS	42.7	46.3	41.2	43.5	.024
RWBS	41.3	47.5	38.9	41.9	.001
PVS	7.0	7.4	6.6	8.4	.692

Note. Income coded 0 thru 5 with 0 = $0-$9,999, 1 = $10,000-$19,999, and 2 = $20,000-$29,999. Time is coded 0 thru 5 with 0 = <1 month, 1 = 1 to 3 months, and 2 = 4 to 6 months.

This result is consistent with Dutton's (1995) findings, which concluded that the greatest contribution to wife assaultive behavior was the childhood victimization of violent men and their feelings of rejection by parental figures in their early developmental years. Although the men in this study tended to use violence when they experienced Orphan energy, it is important to note that it will be impossible for these men, or anyone, to experience true wholeness without incorporating the Orphan. Pearson (1991) explained that initially accepting the shadow side of archetypal energy may cause people to feel less virtuous, but in the long-term it will help them to be more flexible and less one-dimensional.

Table 3 shows the results of the analysis of variance (ANOVA) that was used to test the study hypotheses. The first hypothesis was that European Americans would be more aware of ego level spiritual (archetypal) energy than African Americans. The data (Table 3) showed that there was no significant difference in the awareness of the spiritual (archetypal) energies at the ego development level across ethnic groups. All of the participants scored in the low and mid-range on the ego level archetypal scales. Thus, it appears that the participants were either ambivalent toward embracing spiritual energies at the ego level or they repressed the energy to the extent that it was now controlling them as a shadow.

The second hypothesis, which was that African Americans would show more growth at the soul and spirit levels of development, was supported by the data (Table 3). Growth at the soul level was based upon the degree to which the participants were aware of their purpose in life or reason for existing (EWBS). Growth at the spirit level was measured by the amount of connection the participants had with God or a divine being (RWBS). At both of the aforementioned levels, African Americans had significantly higher scores than the other ethnic groups. These findings support what other ethnically sensitive writers have concluded about spirituality and the awareness of a divine being having paramount importance to the perspective and worldview of African Americans (Kamya, 1997; Schiele, 1996).

CONCLUSIONS

Although this study provides valuable insight into the spiritual development of violent men, it also has limitations. For instance, the generalizability of this study is limited due to the use of a convenience sample of violent men who were in treatment. Thus, these results may not apply to all violent men. Also the reliability of the Innocent (alpha .56) and the Warrior (alpha .63) scales indicates that more modifications are needed to these scales before they can be effectively used in treatment.

Despite these limitations, this study has provided empirical data for an area of practice that continues to be negated and ignored. As such, this can serve as a springboard for incorporating spiritual and religious issues into clinical practice by providing an objective means for understanding and measuring spiritual development in violent men and other clients.

This study introduces a paradigm shift for understanding and treating violent men. The data in this study revealed that certain spiritual forces were significant to the occurrence of physical violence among the men who participated in this study. It also showed that these men, regardless of their ethnic identity, sought to experience spiritual development at three different levels of consciousness: ego, soul, and spirit. Consequently, it is imperative for clients and clinicians to recognize that everyone is a compilation of various spiritual energies that promote multiple perspectives. Thus, a goal of treatment is to value all that makes one who he or she really is, not just who one thinks he or she is. Williams (1998) concluded that more could be accomplished in treatment by healing African American men and teaching them to live a balanced life, rather than by focusing on changing individual behavioral problems (p. 88).

The data showed that African American men in this study, more than other ethnic groups, tended to view the world from the soul and spirit perspectives (Table 3). As such, they are more inclined to view their individual survival as being connected with the collective society (Schiele, 1996; Washburn, 1995). They also tend to seek their divine purpose in life and acknowledge the link that exists between humanity and the universe (Kamya, 1997). This study supports the contention that practitioners who treat African American violent men should consider their spiritual perspective in treatment. Failure to acknowledge this could hamper a clinician's ability to holistically understand their clients' needs.

This study was formulated utilizing a psycho-spiritual theoretical approach that postulates that no one is all good or all bad. One is capable of experiencing spiritual wholeness or completeness when one can acknowledge that one is a compilation of contrasting qualities, such as positive and negative, masculine and feminine, strengths and weaknesses. People often enter therapeutic relationships in search of healing and for reconciliation of the dualism that plagues them. Hammerschlag (1993) said that healing is more than taking care of the mind and body, it is about attending to the damaged spirit. The information derived from this study can aid therapists and social workers in understanding how to do more than impact the mind and body of clients; it will help them to begin touching their souls.

REFERENCES

Asante, M. K. (1988). *Afrocentricity.* Trenton, NJ: African World Press, Inc.

Caplan, R. D., Naidu, R. K., & Tripathi, R. C. (1984). *Journal of Health and Social Behavior, 25,* 303-320.

Carter, C. S. (1999). Church burning in African American communities: Implications for empowerment practice. *Social Work, 44*(1), 62-68.

Clark, M. L., Beckett, J., Wells, M., & Dungee-Anderson, D. (1994). Courtship violence among African American college students. *Journal of Black Psychology, 20*(3), 264-281.

Crandall, J. E., & Rasmussen, R. D. (1975). Purpose in life as related to specific values. *Journal of Clinical Psychology, 31,* 483-485.

Daly, A., Jennings, J., Beckett, J. O., & Leashore, B. R. (1995). Effective coping strategies of African Americans. *Social Work,* 40(2), 240-248.

Dutton, D. (1995). The batterer: A psychological profile. New York: Basic Books.

Ellison, C. W. (1983). Spiritual well-being: Conceptualization and measurement. *Journal of Psychology and Theology, 11*(4), 330-340.

Forte, J. A., Franks, D. D, Forte, J. A., & Rigsby, D. (1996). Asymmetrical role-taking: Comparing battered and nonbattered women. *Social Work, 41*(1), 59-73.

Grove, W. R., Ortega, S. T., & Style, C. B. (1989). The maturational and role perspectives on aging and self through the adult years: An empirical evaluation. *American Journal of Sociology* 94(5), 173-190.

Haight, W. L. (1998). "Gathering the spirit" at First Baptist Church: Spirituality as a protective factor in the lives of African American Children. *Social Work, 43*(3), 213-221.

Hammerschlag, C. A. (1993). *The theft of the spirit.* New York: Simon & Schuster Inc.

Hillman, J. (1972). *The myth of analysis.* Evanston, IL: Northwestern University Press.

Hillman, J. (1975). *Re-visioning psychology.* New York: Harper-Collins.

Hillman, J. (1992). *Soul and spirit.* Common Boundary (November/December), 32-33.

Joseph, M. V. (1987). The religious and spiritual aspects of clinical practice: A neglected dimension of social work. *Social Thought,* (13), 12-23.

Jung, C. G. (1959). *The archetypes and the collective unconscious.* Princeton, NJ: Princeton University Press.

Kamya, H. A. (1997). African immigrants in the United States: The challenge for research and practice. *Social Work, 42*(2), 154-165.

Magruder-Habid, K., Durand, A., & Frey, K. (1991). Alcohol abuse and alcoholism in primary health care settings. *Journal of Family Practice, 32*(4), 406-412.

O'Leary, D. K. (1999). Tailoring interventions to meet the needs of partner abuse clients. *Joining Forces, 3*(3), 1-4.

Paymar, M. (1993). *Violent no more: Helping men end domestic abuse.* Alameda, CA: Hunter House Inc.

Pearson, C. (1991). *Awakening the heroes within: Twelve archetypes to help us find ourselves and transform our world.* New York: HarperCollins Publishing.

Rasheed, J. M., & Rasheed, M. N. (1999). *Social work practice with African American men.* Thousand Oaks, CA: Sage.

Reese, D. J., Ahern, R. E., Nair, S., O'Faire, J. D., & Warren, C. (1999). Hospice access and use by African Americans: Addressing cultural and institutional barriers through participatory action research. *Social Work, 44*(6), 549-559.

Roberts, S. C. (1992). The soul of the world: Exploring archetypal psychology. *Common Boundary*, (November/December), 21-25.

Schiele, J. H. (1996). Afrocentricity: An emerging paradigm in social work practice. *Social Work 41*(3), 284-294.

Singer, J. (1994). *Boundaries of the soul: The practice of Jung's psychology.* Northvale, NJ: Jason Aronson Inc.

Smith, C. D. (1990). *Jung's quest for wholeness: A religious and historical perspective.* Albany: State University of New York Press.

Straus, M. A., & Gelles, R. J. (1990). *Physical violence in American families: Risk factors and adaptations in 8,145 families.* New Brunswick, NJ: Transaction Publishers.

Swigonski, M. E. (1996). Challenging privilege through Africentric social work practice. *Social Work, 41*(2), 153-161.

Warfield-Coppock, N. (1995). Toward a theory of afrocentricity organizations. *Journal of Black Psychology, 21*(1), 30-48.

Washburn, M. (1995). *The ego and the dynamic ground.* New York: State University of New York Press.

Williams, O. J. (1998). Healing and confronting the African American male who batters. In R. Carillo & J. Tello (Eds.), *Family violence and men of color* (pp. 74-94). New York: Springer.

Vanzant, I. (1996). *The spirit of a man: A vision of transformation for black men and the women who love them.* New York: HarperCollins.

Vaughan, F. E. (1991). Spiritual issues in psychotherapy. *Journal of Transpersonal Psychology, 23*(2), 105-119.

Transcending Through Disability and Death: Transpersonal Themes in Living with Cystic Fibrosis

Edward R. Canda

SUMMARY. This study examines transpersonal themes related to a sense of dealing with spiritual transcendence through disability and death as represented in the views of adults with cystic fibrosis (CF), a life threatening chronic hereditary disease. Analysis of on-line discussion, autobiographical writings, and interviews of 16 people with CF identified spiritual

---

Edward R. Canda, PhD, is Professor and Chairperson of the doctoral program at the University of Kansas School of Social Welfare, Lawrence, KS 66045 (E-mail: edc@ukans.edu).

Thanks are due to the following persons: Robert C. Stern, MD, and Carl F. Doershuk, MD, Department of Pediatrics, Case Western Reserve University and Rainbow Babies and Children's Hospital, Cleveland, OH, for crucial assistance at all stages of the research; Ms. Lisa McDonough, columnist for *CF Roundtable,* for generous time and insights about the findings and significance of the study; Paula K. Duke, MA, for going beyond the call of duty as a research assistant. This study was funded in part by the Graduate Research Fund for faculty development through the University of Kansas School of Social Welfare.

This article is dedicated to the memory of Lisa McDonough, who died as it was going to press. In consulting for this study, she became a source of inspiration and friendship for me, as she had for many others through her kind heart and deep insight. She demonstrated that both living and dying can be occasions for spiritual growth and transcendence.

[Haworth co-indexing entry note]: "Transcending Through Disability and Death: Transpersonal Themes in Living with Cystic Fibrosis." Canda, Edward R. Co-published simultaneously in *Social Thought* (The Haworth Press, Inc.) Vol. 20, No. 1/2, 2001, pp. 109-134; and: *Transpersonal Perspectives on Spirituality in Social Work* (ed: Edward R. Canda, and Elizabeth D. Smith) The Haworth Press, Inc., 2001, pp. 109-134. Single or multiple copies of this article are available for a fee from The Haworth Document Delivery Service [1-800-342-9678, 9:00 a.m. - 5:00 p.m. (EST). E-mail address: getinfo@haworthpressinc.com].

beliefs, spiritual metaphors, transpersonal developmental patterns, and accounts of transpersonal experiences, such as miracles and contact with sacred beings. The principles of empowerment and phenomenologically oriented research for transpersonal topics shaped the methodology of this qualitative study. Implications for spiritually sensitive social work practice with people with chronic illnesses are presented. *[Article copies available for a fee from The Haworth Document Delivery Service: 1-800-342-9678. E-mail address: <getinfo@haworthpressinc.com> Website: <http://www.HaworthPress. com> © 2001 by The Haworth Press, Inc. All rights reserved.]*

KEYWORDS. Transpersonal, illness, disability, cystic fibrosis, social work

Hundreds of studies have accumulated in health, mental health, and social work literature on the ways that religious and nonreligious spiritual beliefs and practices contribute to resilience for people with illnesses, disabilities, and other adversities (e.g., Aguilar, 1997; Beckerman & Rock, 1996; Berland, 1995; Canda, Nakashima, Burgess, & Russel, 1999; Dossey, 1993; Dunbar, Mueller, Medina, & Wolf, 1998; Fewell & Vadasy, 1986; Hawks, Hull, Thalman & Richins, 1995; Matthews, Larson, & Barry, 1993; McMillen, 1999; Saleebey, 1997; Sidell, 1997; Turnbull et al., 1993; Young & McNicoll, 1998). These studies have examined the physical and psychosocial benefits provided by personal practices of prayer, meditation, and alternative medical treatments; the social and logistical support given by members of religious communities; and people's efforts to construct a sense of meaning and hope in the midst of chronic distress and crisis. These studies suggest that people's self-care (both conventional medical and alternative), community support, compliance with medical treatments, and self-understanding can all be enhanced by a person's consistent spiritual search for a sense of meaning and purpose as well as particular religious practices and beliefs.

Within social work, several writers have begun to use a transpersonal theoretical perspective to help people deal with crises and illnesses as means of spiritual transformation and growth (Canda & Furman, 1999; Cowley, 1996; Early, 1998; Robbins, Chatterjee, & Canda, 1998; Smith, 1995a & b; Smith, Stefanek, Joseph, & Verdiek, 1993). These theoretical and empirical studies suggest that people's sense of well-being may be enhanced through direct experiences of and beliefs in a transpersonal realm, i.e., enhanced states of consciousness, divine beings, and sacred energies for healing that transcend the ordinary limitations of body, personal ego, linear time, and three dimensional space. All of the studies cited share a common insight that people's resiliency is supported as they weave narratives of learning, unfolding wisdom, and transcendence of mortal limits through their confrontation with illness and disability.

Cystic fibrosis has rarely been addressed explicitly within social work literature. In the only two published empirical studies (Coady, Kent, & Davis, 1990; Driscoll & Lubin,1972), topics of resiliency, spirituality, or views of people with CF were not addressed. An unpublished exploratory interview study of six adults with CF (Cherik, 1999) focused on experiences of grief and loss in relation to chronic illness and how participants supported coping, resilience, and learning. Cherik gave several examples of how various participants used spiritual beliefs and practices (religious and nonreligious) to accept having CF, enhance a sense of closeness with God and other people, support a feeling of mission or divine plan for one's career and life, question deeply the reason for suffering, and convey a feeling of peace. Robbins, Chatterjee, and Canda (1998) used the situation of people with CF to illustrate a way of integrating insights from various theories of human behavior to provide social work practice that addresses physical, mental, social, spiritual, and planetary ecological systems issues. Although this illustration was broad and speculative, it offered theoretical support for the importance of addressing intrapersonal, interpersonal, and cosmic aspects of spirituality in practice with people who have CF.

The present study builds on earlier work to produce a detailed portrait of ways that adults with a life threatening chronic illness, CF, utilize transpersonal beliefs and experiences to achieve a sense of transcendence by working through experience of disability and death. The situation of people with CF serves as an especially strong example of how spirituality can be a resource for resilience in adverse circumstances, since the illness is presently incurable. Presentation of methodology and results will be augmented by biographical and autobiographical accounts of people with CF that elucidate the themes of this study. In addition, conventional academic writing style of third person (i.e., "the author believes . . . ") will be supplemented by first person (i.e., "I" believe . . .) so that the personal qualities of participants' narratives are conveyed realistically.

BIOGRAPHICAL INSIGHTS ON CF AND TRANSFORMATION

Frederick Chopin is commonly regarded as one of the greatest composers for piano. He died at the age of 39 after many years of struggle with chronic respiratory and digestive illnesses, probably due to cystic fibrosis (O'Shea, 1990). Music historians often comment that Chopin's brilliant music is touched with qualities of passion, pathos, and delicateness, perhaps influenced by the challenges of chronic illness.

Chopin's music resounds with the message that illness is an opportunity for wellness and creativity, if people choose to approach it that way. But making the choice to use illness for personal transformation requires courage, perseverance, and spiritual sophistication. It is all too easy for people to feel worn down by illness and thoughts of mortality. But when we make the choice for wellness, we can find many spiritually-based helping and healing activities and support systems that promote physical health and overall well-being. As McDonough (1997), a columnist on CF and spirituality who served as consultant for this study, said, "His life [Chopin's] becomes not a tragedy, but a celebration. Now, whenever I hear his music, I hear the drama, both the angst and the triumph, and tremendous passion" (p. 17).

For the spiritually committed person, struggle with the challenges of CF can become a process of working out theodicy in action. Theodicy literally means "to justify God." In theological terms, it refers to the attempt to make sense out of suffering and to resolve the question of why God would allow it. A Lutheran seminarian with CF, Bill Williams (Williams & Williams, 1998), wove his life experience and theological questioning into a fictionalized novel inspired by the New Testament. The character "jesus" in his book has this to say:

> Imagine being intimately connected with every single thing in the Universe. To know it, feel its needs. To hear the prayer of the sparrow, the ache of a vine, the confusion of a cancer cell. That's one kind of God's power: to be infinitely influenced by the longings of Creation. Now imagine being able to whisper to everything in the Universe. To suggest a tree to the sparrow, a direction to the vine, a protein to the cancer. To lure the world out of senselessness with a vision of the future; to shape it, not by force, but with dreams and compassion. (p. 130)

For some people with CF, the spiritual path is one of examining self, spiritual powers, and one's place in the universe. Canda, another person with CF, summarized it like this:

> Among the symptoms are constant infections and congestion of the lungs, low level fevers, sporadic hemoptysis (coughing up of blood) and the general shortness of breath and vitality. The pancreas is also affected, making digestion problematic. . . . (Yet) sometimes I thank the Lord for CF. There are times when the positive thought comes to mind, "What if I were born Tom but without cystic fibrosis?" I believe the answer to that question would be that I would nearly be a total loss. I believe that CF has made me angry enough to demand some tough answers. (Canda, T., 1987, p. 5)

Wood (1998) explained:

> So how does God turn a horrible disease into something that could shape a life–my life, your life–for His purpose, His glory and our good. . . . How we respond to suffering makes all the difference. Most would say that pain and suffering should be avoided at all costs, but I believe that by handling it correctly, it can be a teacher to lead us into being people of better character. We need to ask ourselves, "Do we want to let this make us bitter or better?" . . . I can honestly say that I am thankful to God because He has used it (CF) to shape me into the person I am . . . am becoming. (p. 10)

Lab described an insight gleaned from his neighbor's avid gardening (Lab & Lab, 1990). He said, "Now my body didn't seem too different from that garden. Nature might not have given me the best stuff to work with, but with care and love and encouragement from the people around me, I seemed to be making it" (p. 71). Stuckert put it this way:

> Choosing to deal with cystic fibrosis, one can find positive attributes that outweigh the hardships involved. From this, we seem to develop an acute awareness and sensitivity to our lives and to life around us. With the realization that our lives may be shorter, we can seek opportunities to enhance the quality of our lives. (quoted in Lab & Lab, 1990, p. 146)

Through our cosmic questions and down to earth answers, a story of spiritual transformation unfolds. McDonough (1998) said:

> What has also become healing for me is to realize that our bodies are not objects, but ongoing stories. In fact, our bodies *are* the story . . . What happens to us comes from our bodies . . . The flesh is the timeline of the soul, its companion, not its competitor. Every one of us is a walking story, unfolding with the narrative drum of heartbeat and blood and cellular respiration . . . Our story isn't over until the last curtain of breath, and even then, our bodies become part of the bigger story of earth and sky, sea and garden. What can make owning or finding our story difficult is when CF is perceived only as a tragedy, rather than an opportunity or a process of discovery. (p. 6)

METHODOLOGY

Paradigm for Inquiry

The heuristic paradigm for social work inquiry shaped this study (Tyson, 1995). In this paradigm, priority is placed on using multiple ways of knowing, perspectives, and types of data in order to construct a holistic and contextual understanding of phenomena. Selection and combination of particular methods are determined by their usefulness for studying the chosen phenomenon. In this study, the focus is on spirituality in a broad sense, referring to a person's search for a sense of meaning, purpose, and morally fulfilling relationships with self, other people, the universe, and the ultimate ground of reality, however understood (Canda, 1997). Therefore, qualitative methods were chosen to explore the subjective understanding of participants' spiritual beliefs and practices and related transpersonal experiences as relevant to dealing with CF. Since transpersonal experiences include phenomena that cannot be directly observed or measured by outside observers (such as supernatural beings and inner mystical visions), qualitative interview methods tapped participants' descriptions of transpersonal experiences and identified patterns among themes within these descriptions (Braud & Anderson, 1998). This heuristic, qualitative approach was coupled with empowerment-oriented research strategies that place a priority on participant involvement in every phase of study in order to ensure that the study directly represented the perspectives of adults with CF and that they benefited from it (Chesler, 1991; Lincoln, 1995; Rapp, Shera, & Kisthardt, 1993). Participants benefited directly through opportunity for self-reflection, referral to support resources, and sharing of findings, and indirectly, through use of findings for information and advocacy for enhanced services for people with CF. The author of this study is also a person with CF. The author's role in carrying out the study and incorporating personal experience as an interviewee ensured an emic (insider's) perspective and phenomenological realism (Braud & Anderson, 1998).

This study's paradigm and methods are consistent with a growing trend in health research that uses qualitative methods to explore issues of meaning and wellness in the midst of illness (Chamberlain, Stephens, & Lyons, 1997; Lincoln, 1992; Loomis, 1997; Maram, 1999; Stephens & Lyons, 1997).

Methods

The author reviewed archived texts from one year of discussion on the Cystic-L on-line group, articles in the mutual support newsletter *CF Roundtable,* books about the lives of people with CF (Deford, 1983; Grishaw, 1995; Lab & Lab, 1990; Staunton, 1991; Woodson, 1991), and personal life experiences in order to develop semi-structured interview questions. In the next stage, 16 adult respondents were identified from the patient population of a national CF treatment center with the help of two physicians (see acknowledgment). A previous quantitative survey at this CF treatment center of all its 402 patients revealed use of spiritually based healing activities (e.g., group prayer, faith healing, use of religious healing objects, religious pilgrimage, meditation, consulting a shaman, and seeking astrological advice) among approximately 60% of patients. However, this survey did not give details of the performance, meaning, and impact of these activities (Stern, Canda, & Doershuk, 1992). The 16 participants (including this author) were selected to reflect a high level of interest in spirituality and a variety of demographic characteristics (see Table 1). This group served as consultants on their own experience and insights and provided suggestions for social workers and health care professionals.

Fifteen respondents were mailed a list of interview topics prior to the interview so they could prepare responses. Topics included the meaning of spirituality and related terms, impact of illness on daily living, use of spiritual activities and supports to deal with CF, and advice for professional helpers. Their telephone interviews (1 1/2-2 hours) were transcribed verbatim and coded, sorted, and analyzed, by the constant comparative method, for patterns

TABLE 1. Participants' Demographic Characteristics

16 Participants:	Including one as researcher
Gender:	8 females; 8 males
Age:	Range from 22-45; including 20s = 4, 30s = 9, 40s = 3
Ethnicity:	2 African American; 14 European American
Religion:	6 Protestant (mainline denominations); 6 Protestant (evangelical, conservative, nondenominational); 2 Catholic; 1 Catholic/Buddhist; 1 Agnostic
Education:	1 less than high school; 3 high school; 11 college degreed; 1 doctorate
Marital/Living Status:	6 married, living with spouse 3 married, living with spouse and children 2 single, living alone 2 separated, living with children 2 single, living with parents or fiancé 1 separated, living alone
Geographic Regions:	14 in 5 mid-western states 2 in 2 southern states
Work Status:	10 full time employed outside home 3 full time homemakers 2 students 1 unemployed
Health Status:	Mild symptoms (less than 1 hospitalization or home I-V antibiotic treatments per year) = 6 Moderate symptoms (1-2 hospitalizations or home I-V treatments per year) = 6 Severe symptoms (3 or more hospitalizations or home I-V treatments per year = 3 Post lung transplant = 1

of themes and variations within themes with the assistance of cut, paste, and sorting features of the MS-Word word-processing program (Berg, 1997; Erlandson, 1993; Lincoln & Guba, 1985; Marshall & Rossman, 1999).

In order to keep interviews focused on the speakers' own life stories. None of these interviewees were informed of the author's personal situation until after interviews were completed, he author used personal experience and study of CF and spirituality to enhance empathic interviewing and to deepen nuances in analysis of data and development of implications. In addition, a trained assistant interviewed the author (for 3 hours) according to the standard interview guide. The resulting transcript was set aside until after all other transcripts were analyzed to reveal themes in an inductive manner with personal assumptions bracketed. This transcript became an external document that allowed the author to take a fresh perspective on personal experience. The results of analyzing this transcript were compared with those of the other 15 interviews. This procedure was helpful to test the breadth of relevance of conclusions, because the author has a significantly different vantage point from the other participants by virtue of his role as researcher as well as unusual features of spiritual perspective and health status.

The themes that emerged from analysis of the first 15 participants were supported through this comparison. Credibility (the faithfulness of researchers' representation of participants' views) was enhanced by feedback from participants in response to a summary of findings as well as a realistic perspective based on the author's personal experience of CF. Transferability of relevance of findings to other people with CF was supported by soliciting reaction to a summary statement from hundreds of participants in the US Adult Cystic Fibrosis Association (Canda, 1999) and two internet based discussion groups for people with CF. All responses were supportive; none contradicted the findings.

In addition, detailed reports of methodology and findings were shared with Ms. Lisa McDonough, a consultant with CF, who is columnist on topics of spirituality and creativity for *CF Roundtable*. She had no involvement with the design of the study or prior contact with the researcher. Two physicians (see acknowledgments) who specialize in treating people with CF served as consultants in order to provide access to participants and medical expertise. Feedback from these three sources also supported the relevance of themes and implications for professional helpers. Credibility and dependability (consistency and effectiveness of research tools and techniques) were supported further through use of a research audit trail and peer review.

In the following presentation of findings, quotation marks represent exact quotes or close paraphrases from respondents' interview transcripts.

Summary of Findings

Spiritual Propensity, Spiritual Imagery, and Transcendence

None of the selection criteria for variation among participants yielded no-
ticeable consistently related patterns of contrast in themes. However, two contrasting groups were discernable based on spiritual propensity. Spiritual
propensity refers to matters of style, perspective, and intensity of belief and
participation in spiritual groups (Canda & Furman, 1999). The two groups'
differences involved variations in the ways that transpersonal experiences and
beliefs were described typically. The first group (n = 6) included exclusively
committed Christians who belong to theologically conservative Protestant denominations (such as Baptist) and non-mainline small church communities.
They identified themselves as born-again Bible-based Christians. They
seemed to have an extrinsic religious orientation. This means that descriptions
of their daily life emphasized frequent participation in religious community
meetings and religious activities at home that were defined largely by the
teachings and norms of their religious group. There was also a high degree of
overlap of social relations between their family members, friends, and religious group members. They indicated a high level of satisfaction with their religious groups and did not indicate any ambiguity or doubt about their
teachings. It should be noted, however, that this did not involve simple confor-
mity or superficial adherence to religious forms. Participants in this group
worked hard to integrate religious teachings and practices into daily life and to
tailor their application to dealing with CF.

Spiritual imagery for this group involved explicit religious references to
their experience of having CF in relation to a struggle between personified supernatural forces. Forces of sacred goodness (Jesus, God, and angels) fought
against demonic forces (Satan, the devil). They described that the devil uses
CF as a weapon of spiritual attack to raise doubts of faith and feelings of dis-
couragement. However, the conservative Christians felt a strong conviction
that they were guaranteed "victory in Christ" over the "trials and tribulations"
caused by the evil forces. In particular instances, they described times when
prayer and support from religious community members helped them to overcome exacerbations of illness and feelings of doubt and despair. Overall, they
said that human mortality and suffering, including the limitations and suffering imposed by CF, would be vanquished ultimately through death, which
their faith transforms into an opportunity for liberation from the body and for
continued existence in heaven in the company of deceased loved ones.

The second group (n = 10) consisted of persons who participate in mainline
Protestant (e.g., Methodist or Lutheran) and Catholic denominations, are more

liberal theologically, and indicate explicit appreciation for other Christian and/or non-Christian spiritual paths. They seemed to have a more intrinsic religious style of spiritual propensity, that is, they were more self-determined, flexible, and constructively critical. For example, one of these self-identified as an agnostic former-Catholic, but she participated in her husband's Protestant church services in order to be supportive. She described her spiritual path as one of enjoying communion with nature and the universe and sharing a sense of "brotherhood with all people." Another is a Protestant married to a Catholic. He and his wife participate in each other's worship services. A third person is a Catholic who practices Zen meditation and studies and participates in many different religious traditions. They shared use of Christian teachings and religious groups with the conservative Christians. However, they also exhibited more questioning and critique of these religious forms, appreciation for other spiritual ways, and flexibility in tailoring their personal spiritual paths in ways that might be unconventional within their primary denominational affiliations. Participants in this group, like the first, worked to integrate religious teachings and practices into daily life and into dealing with CF.

Spiritual imagery varied within this group, with some relying on religious metaphors or broader existential non-religious references. All but the agnostic used Christian theological and biblical references to describe their dealing with CF, just as the first group. They also referred to their relationship with Jesus and God as close and personal. The suffering and challenges of having CF were described in spiritual terms, such as "God created this disease to see what we could do with it and learn from it," or "CF is a very stern teacher about the nature of human life and spiritual potential," or "having CF makes me feel like a survivor of the holocaust," that is, always trying to find ways to survive and find meaning in the midst of suffering. One person referred to Satan but tempered this with a positive spiritual aspect of CF. Helen (participant names are fictitious) said that "CF is one of Satan's warriors" and that Satan would eventually send death "to finish me off." Like the conservative Christians, she said that Christ fights for her against Satan's onslaughts. Paradoxically, she felt that "CF is my closest link to God" because it always reminds her to stay focused on God as a support for her health. And as God helps her to find strength and resilience, she is reminded of God's love for her. Because of God, even death will be a "cleansing" of mortality and suffering that will bring her even closer to God. Most of these ecumenical participants shared the first group's belief that an after-death existence in heaven would afford freedom from limits of the body and a communion of the soul with God.

These two groups have some contrasting uses of spiritual imagery and propensity. However, they share an underlying theme that spiritual beliefs, experiences, and community supports help them to transform their experience of

CF from a merely physical disability into an opportunity for spiritual growth. Indeed, spiritual powers and insights give them the strength to endure and to find meaning within the life challenges of CF. They experience times when sickness and suffering are transformed into occasions of spiritual insight and healing. In their accounts, the constraints of the body and weaknesses of the limited personal ego are transcended, even after death. Even in terms of spiritual imagery, the contrasts between groups are a matter of different emphasis rather than opposition.

Transpersonally Oriented Healing Practices

All 16 participants reported using a variety of transpersonally oriented healing practices as a supplement to conventional medicine. This means that they employed a way of life and specific techniques that tap spiritual resources for healing that they believed exceed ordinary body-ego based capabilities of themselves and loved ones. They relied on power coming from a divine or transcendent source.

Everyone reported some type of benefits to themselves and/or loved ones, though no one claimed to have experienced a cure for CF. Most people used combinations of healing prayer, participation in religious groups, and inspirational reading in the context of a way of life based on faith and a personal relationship or communion with a Sacred Source of power (i.e., God, Jesus, and angels for the Christians; these and Nature and the Universe for the Catholic Zen practitioner; and Nature and the Universe for the agnostic). A few people used a much wider range of healing activities based on a variety of religious and nonreligious traditions and many modes of activity (e.g., diverse states of consciousness, spiritual disciplines, and music). Table 2 summarizes the types of activities and the effects that people most often reported. There was no independent measure of effectiveness. However, it was clear that all participants believed that there were both immediate and long term benefits to themselves and their loved ones through these activities.

A Transpersonal Developmental Path

Although there were many variations among participants regarding the onset, course, and severity of illness, there was a high level of commonality regarding their overall view of personal development. Symptoms associated with CF began during childhood and intensified in severity over time. Periods of relatively good physical health alternated with medical crises, which necessitated hospitalizations and intensive home therapies. Over time, the frequency of medical crises increased as well as the requirements for daily treatments such as antibiotics, pancreatic enzyme supplements, and respiratory clearance

TABLE 2. Types of Transpersonally Oriented Healing Activities

Types	Number Reporting	Typical Effects Reported
Having Faith and Relating with a Sacred Source of Power (e.g. God, Jesus, Angels, Nature, the Universe)	16	Promotes overall well-being and health, sense of meaning and purpose, and yields promise of heavenly after-life.
Healing Prayer (performed by self, loved ones, and religious groups)	13	Decreases illness symptoms; enhances efficacy and endurance of medical treatments; promotes personal qualities of perseverance, joy, hope, peace, encouragement; fosters empathy and intimacy with others; gives sense of meaning and divine protection.

Types	Number Reporting	Typical Effects Reported
Religious Group Activities of Worship and Fellowship	13	Promotes intellectual stimulation, feelings of love and support; reduces depression; encourages openness to others and mutual support; reduces family anxiety; provides material help; stimulates reflection on faith and spirituality; provides benefits under "having faith" and "healing prayer."
Bible Study and Inspirational Reading	10	Decreases symptoms and promotes good self care; provides encouragement, calm, guidance; reduces anxiety; gives insight into social relationships.

Types	Number Reporting	Typical Effects Reported
Use of Spiritual Articles (medals, mementos, sacred herbs, and power objects)	3	Reduces anxiety; reduces symptoms; reminds one to think about life, to pay attention, and to be in harmony.
Communing with Nature	2	Opens healing from earth energy; relieves distress and promotes acceptance; expands sense of oneness and sacredness.
Religious Pilgrimage (by parents or self)	2	Possibly prevents worse symptoms; accesses healing energy from sacred sites; promotes overall well-being.
Listening to Sacred or Inspiring Music	2	Relaxes the body; promotes peacefulness and encouragement.

TABLE 2 (continued)

Types	Number Reporting	Typical Effects Reported
Healing Use of Breathing and Visualization Exercises	2	Eases the lungs and body; relieves strain of coughing; stimulates healing energy; eases distress; invigorates; opens awareness of divine.
Meditation and Mantra Practice	1	Relieves distress; enhances work performance; promotes clarity, awareness of divine, and preparation for death.
Meditative Massage/Accupressure	1	Relieves bodily strain; reduces symptoms; reduces distress.
Christian Counseling	1	Promotes self-acceptance; reduces anger; improves family relations; promotes search for meaning.
Meditative Group Drumming	1	Stimulates healing energy; prevents illnesses; invigorates body; relieves distress; encourages mutual support; promotes clarity and insight.

therapies. Participants anticipated progression of the illness to a so-called "end-stage," meaning a health condition so critical that death would result without a lung transplant.

These physical challenges might seem to paint a bleak picture. However, participants told a different story. Chronic physical illness created a challenge to understand why this was happening. Many described themselves as having been precociously interested in the meaning and purpose of life because of health challenges and awareness of mortality. Keen awareness of mortality also heightened participants' commitment to high quality social relationships, appreciation for life, and using opportunities to help themselves and to draw others closer to God or other notions of a sacred Higher Power (such as nature or ultimate oneness of the universe). Thus, as participants' physical condition worsened, their sense of overall personal well-being and spiritual vitality increased. This insight is reinforced by the observation of the single participant who had a lung transplant. She said that it was ironic that while she had severe symptoms of CF, she had the benefit of being constantly reminded to attend to her spiritual life. But after the transplant, her new sense of comfort led her to be more complaisant.

This is not to say that this developmental path is an easy one. Everyone described times of great physical discomfort, emotional stress, intellectual quandary, and social relational impediment. Two participants described themselves as often overwhelmed by the distresses of having CF. However, they recognized that they were on a path of spiritual transformation. Further, participants' descriptions of variations of temporary attitude (such as despondence or optimism) did not relate consistently to demographic characteristics or severity of illness.

For most participants, death itself was not perceived as a dead end. Participants were not asked directly about their feelings regarding death, since this might have posed too great discomfort. Yet fourteen of the 16 people brought up the subject. Five people emphasized the difficulty of dealing with mortality and death, because of the danger of dying young and uncomfortably, the desire to enjoy a long life with family and loved ones, and fear of the unknown.

Twelve participants explained that their spiritual orientations mitigated the negative aspects of death. As the conservative Christian participants often put it, they would have victory over CF through Christ, even in death. Twelve participants mentioned that they believed in heaven or some type of after-death existence. This was described as "a magnificent and much better place" (n = 6), "an opportunity to reunite with deceased relatives and loved ones" (n = 5), "freedom from CF" (n = 5), "discovery of the meaning of life" (n = 2), and "the fruit of how one has lived" (n = 1). Eight people said that they looked forward to heaven. Eleven described death as a "transition" or "the last great challenge" for more spiritual growth.

This transformational potential of life and death with CF related to participants' world views. Everyone described some way of blending commitments to cultivate their own spiritual well-being, to serve and inspire other people, and to grow throughout life to be closer to God or their sacred Higher Power. To weave together care of self and others with faith in the divine or the sacredness of existence was the meaning and purpose of life shared by participants.

Transpersonal Experiences

Participants' spiritual beliefs were not simply a matter of intellectual assent to religious creeds or unquestioning belief. Spiritual beliefs were presented as articulations of deep experiences of communion with faith communities and divine transpersonal beings and forces. Twelve participants described miracles or extraordinary events that reaffirmed their beliefs and sustained their physical health and spiritual development (see Table 3). In addition, everyone reported significant experiences of a transpersonal nature, such as feeling a close personal relationship with God or transcending the ordinary limitations of the body and personal ego.

TABLE 3. Transpersonal Experiences Described by Participants

Reporting	Number
Vivid sense of connection with ultimate reality (God, universe)	16
God and Jesus or angelic forces assist the person	15
Prayer or other spiritual forms of healing directly cure or reduce certain symptoms	7
Person senses God conquering devil	7
Prayer leads to correct medical treatment	2
God gives extraordinary strength and endurance during crisis	2
Revelatory dreams or visions occur	2
God's presence is felt intensely	2
Person feels deep sense of communion with nature	2
Deceased brother appears	1
God gives sense of amazing peace and joy	1
God gives extraordinary inspiration through Bible reading	1

The following summaries from two participants' experiences portray transpersonal themes vividly in the context of two people's life details. Joan's story was chosen because of her ability to articulate clearly a wide range of themes on development and transpersonal experiences shared by all participants. The author's story is used to illustrate the theme of transpersonal experiences that support a sense of transcending death. Also, this affords an opportunity to weave self-reflection into this research account, in keeping with phenomenological inquiry. These two stories are examples of contrasting spiritual styles (conservative and ecumenical) that share common themes. Both of us described more accounts of intense transpersonal experiences than other participants.

A Circle of Protection

Joan is a European American, in her 30s, married, and employed full time in a professional career. She is a nondenominational Protestant who regards her personal relationship with God and Jesus as most important in her life. She divided her life development into four phases. During phase 1, early childhood, her symptoms of CF did not significantly impede daily life. During phase 2, from mid childhood to late 20s, symptoms increased in severity, necessitating hospital based treatment (about 2 weeks each) every 1 to 1 1/2 years, plus intensive home treatments on a daily basis. She was able to maintain her daily schedule of activities, including college education and career. However, during her 30s (phase 3), there was a dramatic decline of health, resulting in life threatening illness and need for a lung transplant. In her late 30s, she had a successful lung transplant that dramatically improved her physical health, commencing phase 4.

Joan explained that during phase 2, her trust in God and religious upbringing gave her a sense of hope and the motivation to persevere. But phase 3 presented a harsh challenge:

> That was a very difficult time because everything I had learned up until then with faith and how to cope with my health physically and mentally was just swept totally away . . . Even though I had the spiritual foundation it was shaken like it never was before . . . My body was falling apart around me.

During this time, she relied heavily on "reminders of God's steadfastness" as provided through her childhood religious learning, reading in the Bible, listening to Christian audio tapes, and prayer:

> It felt like I was out over the waters, hanging on to nothing. And God was hanging on to me by the back of my shirt but I couldn't feel that. I was just like aaaah (quiet scream)! I had to have so much trust without any foundation or any physical reason to trust.

When Joan and her husband were waiting for her lung transplant, she felt so ill and weak that she had to give up attachment to life. "I had to really, really in my heart of hearts say, 'Okay, if you (God) want me to die right now, that's okay." She described this as "very much a drawing in. It was like the world went into a tiny little thing, everything drawn in very close. It was like 'Oh, this is how it is to be dying.'"

Although this was a terrible feeling, she recounted many experiences that reassured her of God's supportive presence. She and her husband felt there was a "circle of protection" around her:

> It was an unreal, surreal kind of thing. But it was very comforting, even though there was still anxiety in the midst of that. It was an intensity of experience and emotion and a spiritual closeness to God that I hadn't had before . . . It was the presence, maybe not him (God) himself, but like his protecting, like an angel.

This awareness of an angelic circle of protection opened up through a series of dreams that symbolized both her helpless decline into sickness and death as well as her sustenance by divine powers. In one dream, she and her husband were in the back of a church. Joan was very sick. A cold hard wind began to blow and flap around her. Suddenly, the very strong yet gentle hand of the "angel Michael" grabbed her. The angel and her husband held her so that she would not be blown away. And Joan yelled "at the top of her lungs" the name of Jesus in order to be protected from Satan's harm. Then the angel helped her and her husband to put on rain gear that would be "protection for the times ahead."

This protection stayed with her throughout the times of greatest sickness and transplant. "I can remember that protection feeling, like when we were doing therapies" despite the discomfort and grueling schedule of treatments. This gave a sense of strength to her husband to endure as well:

> We really could feel this supernatural strength that was there that we really didn't have on our own. And that whole feeling lasted all the way up through the transplant. By the time of the transplant, I was totally exhausted, but I was just so ready. There was no real fear there . . . If I died on the table, I said, "That's okay."

And after the transplant,

> that protection was there. I can remember a couple times (even several years) after the transplant, getting this unusually hot feeling in my chest, like a joy . . . This was so weird! Something that lasted a day and a half. You know, I don't really make up things. And I thought, "What is that all about?" But I don't know what it was, almost feel like it'd be the Holy Spirit.

Since the transplant, she has had greatly improved physical health. But she also has had more temptations to be distracted from her spiritual commitments. So she keeps reminding herself to stay on her path. Although she hadn't had the intense feeling of the angelic presence lately, she did continue to feel very comfortable. "I think I've taken away from that whole experience that God is really with me. I am absolutely not afraid of anything physically." She said that although she would be scared and depressed with a new health crisis, "there is such a deep, deep, deep sense of connectedness with God that I don't think will ever go away."

Death as a Continuation of Life

Since the following is based on the author's experience, it is necessary to shift to a first person style of presentation to be realistic. Although this is not common in conventional academic writing, it is consistent with the phenomenological approach of this study.

I am a European American, in my 40s, married, and employed full time as a social work professor. I am a Catholic who practices Zen meditation and incorporates ideas and practices from many religious traditions into my spiritual style. In doing this study, I was inspired by the courage, clarity, and wisdom of the people I interviewed. I was constantly challenged to reflect between other people's accounts of dealing with CF and my own experience, thus engendering my own learning and growth as well as insights into the themes and significance emerging from the study.

During many interviews, especially of conservative Christian participants, I felt great difference from my own rather unconventional worldview and way of thinking about spirituality. In fact, I have incorporated much more variety of religious tradition, spiritual cultivation practice, and alternative healing strategy than have the other participants. Yet throughout all of the interviews, I had a sense of kinship and familiarity that transcended these differences. This connection arose from commonalties in the practical health challenges we all face. But even more deeply, the connection related to the feeling that we all shared a commitment to transform and transcend our experience of illness through life long learning, soul searching, and practices designed to cultivate a profound relationship between ourselves, loved ones, the world, and our Sacred Source of strength, however differently we conceived of it.

A portion of my interview referred to the theme of transcending death. Most of the participants addressed this, but my account was the most detailed. In general, I described my involvement with Christian and Buddhist practices of meditation and prayer, as well as various religious teachings on possibilities of an after-death form of life. I described some of my death preparation practices that are intended to optimize the likelihood that I can move through the dying process with clarity. However, I emphasized that for me, it is important to refrain from fixing on any literal view of what happens after death. I would rather be open to mystery. My main point was that by dealing with the opportunities for learning and self-improvement provided by every moment of living and dying, including the challenges of CF, we can be ready to experience death and its aftermath in the best way. Then death becomes one more step in the moment-to-moment process of spiritual transformation.

I recounted some experiences relating to relationship with my brother, Tom, who died from symptoms related to CF at the age of 41. Tom and I had discussed matters of philosophy and spirituality, including speculations about death, ever since our teens. As an older brother, he often learned about such things before me and shared them with me. Also, as his illness symptoms were consistently more severe than mine, I could learn strategies to deal with my illness by observing what did or did not work well for him.

He said that it was important to him that he could play that role, that he felt that was something he could contribute to me; like he was a pioneer going through that first and so then I could maximize my health by learning from him. So in a way I feel like that was a gift from him to me.

Before Tom died:

> he had asked me to take his cremation remains up to the Rocky Mountains and do a ceremony to disperse his ashes . . . When I went out, I selected a spot that was on my friend's land out there, a fairly pristine area, and did a ceremony. And I felt really strongly during that period (of three years) that he (Tom) was present. I felt like he was present in the wind when it blew . . . He liked crows. I'd hear crows or see a crow and I would feel reminded of his presence. It was almost like something of him re-entered the elements of the natural environment. (I felt that way) especially during the three year period when I did ceremonies for him. That was a particularly vivid sense of connection with him, partly because it was helping him in his after-death process, but it was also a feeling of him helping me, like when he was alive, we were brothers helping each other. So sometimes I have that feeling that he is present and supportive. I don't take these things literally or concretely though. I just accept it . . . as a gift.

> One event made this really vivid. When he died, I had just visited him about a week earlier. I went out to Ohio; I had this feeling he would die soon. We had a really nice, very warm and moving time together. When I found out he died, I quickly arranged for a flight out so I'd be there for the memorial service.

> My wife and I were staying in my parents' guest room which is the bedroom where Tom and I used to share. The night before or after the memorial, when I was sleeping, I felt somebody tap my leg. I woke up and saw the presence of my brother kind of hovering above the bed. Not like his literal body, but an amorphous presence that had the feeling tone of my brother; and I just felt from him an affirmation and support of our connection. And that he was okay. And then I fell back to sleep.

> The amazing thing was how matter of fact it was at the time . . . So it went underneath my questioning analytical mind, that might have screened something out, and was just completely ordinary . . . And then later I remembered that when we were younger and we talked about death, we said that whichever of us dies first should come back and give a sign to the other person, you know, that there really is something on the other side. (Chuckle). And (remembering that) I said, "Oh wow! He kept his promise!" So that was pretty cool.

Implications for Spiritually Sensitive Social Work Practice

Aguilar (1997) advocated for a holistic approach to social work in health care that attends to spirituality and transpersonal experiences. In Canda and Furman's (1999) framework, spiritually sensitive practice is founded on values, knowledge, and skills that promote the dignity of all persons and all spiritual paths, religious and nonreligious. They also point out that transpersonal theory and practice approaches can facilitate clients' spiritual development by focusing on ways to assess and encourage life experiences that join the individual in a responsible and edifying way with other people, non-human beings, and the ground of being. However, there are cautions about limitations of transpersonal theory to be considered (Robbins, Chatterjee, & Canda, 1998). This discussion will consider how insights from participants shed light on both the helpful and unhelpful aspects of transpersonal theory for practice.

Of course, the themes identified in this study cannot be generalized in the statistical sense of external validity to all people with CF or other disabilities. However, the techniques for supporting transferability increase confidence that these themes are likely to be shared by other adults with CF for whom faith, religion, and spirituality are highly important. This leads to suggestions for enhancing social work practice for people with CF. A further significance of this study is that it shows that for some people, spirituality can be a tremendous resource for dealing with various kinds of illness and disability. Participants' experiences offer useful suggestions for others with disabilities and chronic illnesses, helping professionals who work with them, and indeed all people, to consider in dealing with human fragility, mortality, and death. This study also lends support to the many studies cited in the introduction indicating that spirituality can be an important resource for resilience for people dealing with adversity.

The plot lines of the participants' stories do not run through a standard set of developmental stages associated with age, cognitive abilities, and social roles, as described in the life span theories of Erikson, Kohlberg, Piaget, Fowler, Jung, and their followers (Robbins, Chatterjee, & Canda, 1998). Even leading transpersonal theorists tend to accept this portrayal of the life span, since they rely heavily on these conventional theorists to describe development of the personal ego (e.g., Washburn, 1995; Wilber, 1995).

In contrast, the participants described their development over the life span in phases that are marked by significant changes impacting physical, mental, social, and spiritual aspects of life. These punctuate the life story. Therefore, the developmental path is not standardized; it is distinctive to each person. Joan's story is a good example of this.

In the physical aspect, participants' life phases relate to such markers as changes in severity of symptoms, time of diagnosis, health crises and resolutions, hospitalizations, and lung transplants. In the mental aspect, participants described challenges to their emotional well-being and intellectual beliefs, which were largely attributed to the physical changes. In the social aspect, the formation of relationships of support with members of the family of origin, spouses, friends, and spiritual support community were important. The nature of these relationships also connected to physical changes and challenges. In the spiritual aspect, all of these fluctuations were given a sense of meaning and significance in relationship with spiritual communities and some belief in and experience of a Sacred Source of strength, which varied with the spiritual perspective.

Since the physical challenges posed questions of meaning and heightened concern about the truth and relevance of religious teachings, participants described spiritual commitments developing often in childhood. These people were exceptions to life span and cognitive stage theorists' standardized schedules, which attribute spiritual preoccupations to middle adulthood and older. Actually, the participants can be described, in Erikson's (1962 & 1969) terms, as *homo religiosi,* Latin for "religious people." By this, Erikson meant people who are precociously and intensely concerned about spiritual matters and guide their life paths toward a sense of personal meaning and social responsibility. It appears that this heightened spiritual interest related to a combination of challenges set by CF early in life, together with the person's choice to approach them as opportunities for growth. Coles' (1990) interviews of children in many cultures demonstrated that this propensity for spiritual reflection may be much more common in youth than life span theories, both conventional and transpersonal, suggest.

This study supports models of human development that are responsive to individual and cultural variations of the life course, unpredictability of life events, capacity for personal choice and creativity, issues of disability, and crisis, resiliency, and transformative possibilities inherent in adversity (Germain, 1991 & 1994). As this study and the literature review indicated, one needs to add the possibility of transpersonal experiences, including spiritual crises and breakthroughs, and the capacity of some people to achieve spiritual growth through creative engagement with adversity.

Canda and Furman's (1999) timeline of spiritual development would likely serve as a more useful tool for assessing people with chronic illness than tools based on standardized life stage models, even those that are oriented transpersonally. It involves discussing the client's life story and collaboratively formulating a timeline of key transitional events (such as health crises or transpersonal experiences) plotted out by days, months, or years, as relevant. The ups, downs, and plateaus of spiritual development can be charted with no presumptions of order or standardization by the social worker. In addition, at each phase demarcated by the client, information can be supplied about relevant spiritual practices used to deal with illness; qualities of spiritual insights about the meaning, purpose, and transformational potential of having a chronic illness; participation in religious or nonreligious support groups, especially regarding impact on health care and its psychosocial aspects; the helpful role of spiritual exemplars, mentors, and friends; and key beliefs, rituals, and symbols that the client has used or wishes to develop in supporting a resilient response to the chronic illness. This need not be done through a linear graphic representation. Children and creative adults may be more inclined to drawing pictures and telling autobiographical stories in a fluid form.

Most research participants stated that they did not view death as the end of the life span. This study shows that for people who believe death is a transition, anticipation of death and the process of dying can be used as further opportunities for developing insight and sense of well being. If social workers are to create developmental models that are congruent with people's beliefs in an after-death life, the conventional developmental theories need to be modified. This is especially important because most Americans believe in an after-life, and, indeed, most religious traditions in the world promote this (Nielsen et al., 1993; Sheridan, Bullis, Adcock, Berlin, & Miller, 1992; Sheridan, Wilmer, & Atcheson, 1994).

It is not necessary for a social worker to agree with any particular belief or to be familiar personally with any particular transpersonal experience of a client. But it is necessary to understand them and to engage them constructively in the helping process. Some religious ideas and transpersonal experiences recounted in this study were not shared by all participants. Some would be different from and even in conflict with many other people's beliefs. But the pattern of support experienced by all participants from some type of transpersonal experiences and religious beliefs shows that the transpersonal realm is of potential benefit to people, albeit in forms that fit the cultural and personal characteristics of each person. Jung's idea of psychic reality (Robbins, Chatterjee, & Canda, 1998) is helpful here. Jung pointed out that an intense transpersonal experience is real *for that person,* and that is where the process of helping must begin. As Canda and Furman (1999) explained, people may change their interpretations of a transpersonal event over time as they practice self-reflection and observe the impact on life circumstances. Indeed, the social worker can help people who have transpersonal experiences sort out the meaning, differentiate from psychopathology, and integrate insights from them into daily life (Nelson, 1994). This process may be especially important for people with chronic illness, because of the higher "stakes" for making sense of life and death in relation to coping with health challenges.

Participant accounts of transpersonal experiences and healing activities support transpersonal theories' interest in these phenomena and their claims that transpersonal experiences can enhance development. A representative national survey of practitioner members of the National Association of Social Workers showed that most social workers do address, and/or believe it is appropriate to address, various types of transpersonal experiences and practices with clients, such as related to prayer, rituals, spiritual self-reflection, dreams, and exploring spiritual meaning of life and death (Canda & Furman, 1999). However, the same survey showed that most social workers feel inadequately educated and prepared to do so. The findings of this study suggest that such educational preparation might be especially important for work with clients with chronic illness who are interested in spirituality.

Many participants pointed out that their particular form of illness is distinctive, but that all people share challenges of illness, mortality, disability, and death at some point. They expressed the hope that their learning from experience might encourage others to appreciate life, to prepare wisely for death, and to clarify the spiritual path that will help them to do so.

REFERENCES

Aguilar, M. A. (1997). Re-engineering social work's approach to holistic healing: Guest editorial. *Health and Social Work, 22*(2), 83-84.

Beckerman, N., & Rock, M. (1996). Themes from the frontlines: Hospital social work with people with AIDS. *Social Work in Health Care, 23*(4), 75-89.

Berg, B. L. (1997). *Qualitative research methods for the social sciences.* Boston: Allyn and Bacon.

Berland, W. (1995). Can the self affect the course of cancer? *Advances: The Journal of Mind-Body Health, 11*(4), 5-19.

Braud, W., & Anderson, R. (1998). *Transpersonal research methods for the social sciences.* Thousand Oaks, CA: Sage.

Bullis, R. K. (1996). *Spirituality in social work practice.* Washington, DC: Taylor & Francis.

Canda, E. R. (1997). Spirituality. In R. L. Edwards (Ed.), *Social work encyclopedia, 19th ed., 1997 Supplement.* Washington, DC: National Association of Social Workers Press.

Canda, E. R. (Ed.). (1998). *Spirituality in social work: New directions.* New York: The Haworth Press, Inc.

Canda, E. R. (1999, Summer). Consensus statement on spirituality by adults with CF. In L. McDonough, Spirit medicine: Declaration of inspiration. *CF Roundtable* (pp. 6-7).

Canda, E. R., & Furman, L. D. (1999). *Spiritual diversity in social work practice: The heart of helping.* New York: The Free Press.

Canda, E. R., Nakashima, M., Burgess, V., & Russel, R. (1999). *Spiritual diversity and social work: A comprehensive bibliography with annotations.* Alexandria, VA: Council on Social Work Education.

Canda, T. P. (1987). A blessing from God. *Inherit the Earth: A Publication of the Catholic Worker Community of Cleveland, 3*(1), 1-6.

Chamberlain, K., Stephens, C., & Lyons, A. C. (1997). Encompassing experience: Meanings and methods in health psychology. *Psychology and Health, 12,* 691-709.

Cherik, L. (1999). *Unacknowledged grief and loss in chronic illness: Identifying grief and loss themes in cystic fibrosis.* Unpublished master's thesis, University of St. Thomas and College of St. Catherine School of Social Work, St. Paul, MN.

Chesler, M. A. (1991). Participatory action research with self-help groups: An alternative paradigm for inquiry and action. *American Journal of Community Psychology, 19*(5), 757-768.

Coady, C. A., Kent, V. D., & Davis, P. W. (1990). Burnout among social workers working with patients with cystic fibrosis. *Health and Social Work, 15*(2), 116-124.

Coles, R. (1990). *The spiritual life of children.* Boston: Houghton Mifflin.

Cowley, A. (1996). Transpersonal social work. In F. J. Turner (Ed.), *Social work treatment: Interlocking theoretical approaches* (4th ed., pp. 663-698). New York: The Free Press.

Deford, F. (1983). *Alex: The life of a child.* Baltimore: Cystic Fibrosis Foundation.

Derezotes, D., & Evans, K. E. (1995). Spirituality and religiosity in practice: In-depth interviews of social work practitioners. *Social Thought, 18*(1), 39-56.

Dossey, L. (1993). *Healing words: The power of prayer and the practice of medicine.* San Francisco: Harper San Francisco.

Driscoll, C. B., & Lubin, A. H. (1972). Conferences with parents of children with cystic fibrosis. *Social Casework, 53*(3), 140-146.

Dudley, J. R., & Helfgott, C. (1990). Exploring a place for spirituality in the social work curriculum. *Journal of Social Work Education, 26*(3), 287-294.

Dunbar, H. T., Mueller, C. W., Medina, C., & Wolf, T. (1998). Psychological and spiritual growth in women living with HIV. *Social Work, 43*(2), 144-154.

Early, B. P. (1998). Between two worlds: The psychospiritual crisis of a dying adolescent. In E. R. Canda (Ed.), *Spirituality in social work: New directions* (pp. 67-80). Binghamton, NY: Haworth Pastoral Press.

Erikson, E. H. (1962). *Young man Luther: A study in psychoanalysis and history.* New York: Norton.

Erikson, E. H. (1969). *Gandhi's truth: On the origins of militant nonviolence.* New York: Norton.

Erlandson, D. A., Harris, E.L., Skipper, B.L., & Allen, S.D. (1993). *Doing naturalistic inquiry.* Newbury Park: Sage.

Fewell, R. R., & Vadasy, P. F. (Eds.). (1986). *Families of handicapped children: Needs and supports across the life span.* Austin, TX: Pro-ed.

Germain, C. B. (1991). *Human behavior in the social environment: An ecological view.* New York: Columbia University Press.

Germain, C. B. (1994). Emerging conceptions of family development over the life course. *Families in Society, 75*(5), 259-267.

Grishaw, J. (1995). *My heart is full of wishes.* Austin, TX: Raintree Steck-Vaughan Publishers.

Hawks, S. R., Hull, M. L., Thalman, R. L., & Richins, P. M. (1995). Review of spiritual health: Definition, role, and intervention strategies in health promotion. *American Journal of Health Promotion, 9*(5), 371-378.

Joseph, M. V. (1987). The religious and spiritual aspects of clinical practice. *Social Thought, 13,* 2-23.

Lab, D., & Lab, O. K. (1990). *My life in my hands: Living with cystic fibrosis.* Thousand Palms, CA: LabPro Press.

Lincoln, Y. S. (1992). Sympathetic connections between qualitative methods and health research. *Qualitative Health Research, 2*(4), 375-391.

Lincoln, Y. S. (1995). Emerging criteria for quality in qualitative and interpretive research. *Qualitative Inquiry, 1*(3), 275-289.

Lincoln, Y., & Guba, E. (1985). *Naturalistic inquiry.* Beverly Hills: Sage.

Loomis, F. L. (1997). Illness as opportunity: Lessons from chronic fatigue. *Reflections: Narratives of Professional Helping, 3*(1), 25-28.

Maram, M. (1999). Breast cancer: A personal and professional crisis. *Reflections: Narratives of Professional Helping, 5*(1), 39-44.

Marshall, C., & Rossman, G. (1999). *Designing qualitative research.* Thousand Oaks, CA: Sage.

Matthews, D. A., Larson, D. B., & Barry, C. P. (1993). *The faith factor: An annotated bibliography of clinical research on spiritual subjects* (Vol. 1). MD: National Institute for Healthcare Research.

McDonough, L. (1997, Spring). Spirit medicine: Guess who else had CF? *CF Roundtable,* 17.

McDonough, L. (1998, Winter). Spirit medicine: The body as story. *CF Roundtable,* 6.

McMillen, J. C. (1999). Better for it: How people benefit from adversity. *Social Work, 44*(5), 455-468.

Nelson, J. E. (1994). *Healing the split: Integrating spirit into our understanding of the mentally ill* (Rev. ed.). Albany: State University of New York Press.

Nielsen, N. C. et al. (1993). *Religions of the world* (3rd ed.). New York: St. Martin's Press.

O'Shea, J. (1990). *Was Mozart poisoned? Medical investigations into the lives of the great composers.* New York: St. Martin's Press.

Rapp, C., Shera, W., & Kisthardt, W. (1993). Research strategies for consumer empowerment of people with severe mental illness. *Social Work, 38*(6), 727-735.

Robbins, S. P., Chatterjee, P., & Canda, E. R. (1998). *Contemporary human behavior theory: A critical perspective for social work.* Boston: Allyn & Bacon.

Saleebey, D. (Ed.). (1997). *The strengths perspective in social work practice* (2nd ed.). New York: Longman.

Sheridan, M. J., Bullis, R. K., Adcock, C. R., Berlin, S. D., & Miller, P. C. (1992). Practitioners' personal and professional attitudes toward religion and spirituality: Issues for education and practice. *Journal of Social Work Education, 28*(2), 190-203.

Sheridan, M. J., Wilmer, C. M., & Atcheson, L. (1994). Inclusion of content on religion and spirituality in the social work curriculum: A study of faculty views. *Journal of Social Work Education, 30*(3), 363-376.

Sidell, N. L. (1997). Adult adjustment to chronic illness: A review of the literature. *Health and Social Work, 22*(1), 5-11.

Siporin, M. (1985). Current social work perspectives on clinical practice. *Clinical Social Work Journal, 13*(3), 198-217.

Smith, E. (1995). Addressing the psychospiritual distress of death as reality: A transpersonal approach. *Social Work, 40,* 402-413.

Smith, E. D., Stefanek, M. E., Joseph, M. V., & Verdieck, M. J. (1993). Spiritual awareness, personal perspective on death and psychosocial distress among cancer patients: An initial investigation. *Journal of Psychosocial Oncology, 11*(3), 89-103.

Staunton, V. (1991). *Gillian: A second chance.* Dublin, Ireland: Blackwater Press.

Stern, R. C., Canda, E. R., & Doershuk, C. F. (1992). Use of nonmedical treatment by cystic fibrosis patients. *Journal of Adolescent Health, 13,* 612-615.

Turnbull, A. P., Patterson, J. M., Behr, S. K., Murphy, D. L., Marquis, J. G., & Blue-Banning, M. J. (1993). *Cognitive coping, families, & disability.* Baltimore: Paul H. Brookes.

Tyson, K. (1995). *New foundations for scientific and behavioral research: The heuristic paradigm.* Boston: Allyn and Bacon.

Washburn, M. (1995). *The ego and the dynamic ground: A transpersonal theory of human development* (2nd ed.). Albany: State University of New York Press.

Wilber, K. (1995). *Sex, ecology, spirituality: The spirit of evolution.* Boston: Shambhala.

Williams, B., & Williams, M. (1998). *Naked before God: The return of a broken disciple.* Harrisburg, PA: Morehouse Publishing.

Wood, L. (1998, Autumn). CF–A chisel to a beautiful life. *CF Roundtable,* 10.

Woodson, M. (1991). *Turn it into glory.* Minneapolis: Bethany House Publishers.

Young, J. Y., & McNicoll, P. (1998). Against all odds: Positive life experiences of people with advanced amyotrophic lateral sclerosis. *Health and Social Work, 23*(1), 35-43.

Addressing Spirituality in Hospice: Current Practices and a Proposed Role for Transpersonal Social Work

Dona J. Reese

SUMMARY. Despite evidence of the importance of spirituality to terminally ill patients, the social work profession has developed few curriculum materials, practice models, or research on this topic. This chapter presents theoretical and empirical support for the proposition that transition to the transegoic stage of consciousness can promote a comfortable death for hospice patients and that hospice social workers should address spiritual issues in order to assist terminally ill patients and their families in making this transition. It also presents the results of a national survey describing and testing the effectiveness of some current social work approaches to addressing spirituality in hospice. Implications for practice and social work education are explored. *[Article copies available for a fee from The Haworth Document Delivery Service: 1-800-342-9678. E-mail address:*

Dona J. Reese, PhD, LCSW, is affiliated with the Social Work Program at the University of Arkansas, 211 Old Main, Fayetteville, AR 72701 (E-mail: reese@mail.uark.edu).

National Hospice Social Work Survey results reported in this article were part of a larger study in which the author served as principal investigator, with coinvestigators Mary Raymer and Joan Richardson. This study was a general survey of the impact of social work services upon client outcomes and was jointly funded by the National Hospice Organization and Hospice of the Florida Suncoast. The author wishes to express appreciation to Henry Hexmoor for help in developing the theoretical basis of this article, and to Linda Lorentz-Dockter, MSW, for help in analyzing the qualitative data.

[Haworth co-indexing entry note]: "Addressing Spirituality in Hospice: Current Practices and a Proposed Role for Transpersonal Social Work." Reese, Dona J. Co-published simultaneously in *Social Thought* (The Haworth Press, Inc.) Vol. 20, No. 1/2, 2001, pp. 135-161; and: *Transpersonal Perspectives on Spirituality in Social Work* (ed: Edward R. Canda, and Elizabeth D. Smith) The Haworth Press, Inc., 2001, pp. 135-161. Single or multiple copies of this article are available for a fee from The Haworth Document Delivery Service [1-800-342-9678, 9:00 a.m. - 5:00 p.m. (EST). E-mail address: getinfo@haworthpressinc.com].

KEYWORDS. Transpersonal, spirituality, hospice, social work, death

Transpersonal social work is a leading practice theory (Canda & Furman, 1999; Smith, 1995) that encompasses spirituality as a universal aspect of human development. As a source of strength for clients, spirituality is an important area of attention in practice. Within the highest stage of consciousness development, the transegoic stage, individuals are able to move beyond a focus on concerns of the separate ego and to develop a holistic sense of union between the Ultimate and the ordinary (Wilber, 1995, 1996). This article proposes that transition to the transegoic stage of consciousness promotes a comfortable death for hospice patients and that use of transpersonal theory by hospice social workers to address spiritual issues can assist terminally ill patients and their families in making this transition. Few social work programs provide training in addressing spiritual issues, however (Quattlebaum & Cascio, 1999). There are few practice models or evaluation studies testing the effectiveness of social work interventions with spirituality. Therefore, this article discusses the use of transpersonal theory as a basis for practice techniques to help people deal with death and dying. It presents the results of a national survey describing and testing the effectiveness of some current social work approaches to addressing spirituality in hospice. Implications for practice and social work education are explored.

A TRANSPERSONAL PERSPECTIVE

Transpersonal Experience and Spirituality

Transpersonal theory as proposed by Wilber (1980, 1993, 1995, 1996) is based on the perspective that human development is a process of evolution in which each person, and the human species as a whole, is developing toward unitary consciousness (Canda & Furman, 1999). Levels of consciousness development as proposed by Wilber include: (a) the preegoic, in infancy and early childhood, in which the child has not yet achieved an awareness of ego separate from the world; (b) the egoic, from older childhood on, in which the individual achieves a clear sense of autonomous ego, ability for rational thought, and mature social relationships; and (c) the transegoic stage, which is normally not achieved until adulthood, and possibly not at all. Individuals do not automatically progress to this last stage, but must engage in spiritual practice, such as meditation, and make deliberate efforts toward functioning at a transegoic level of consciousness. In this stage, the sense of self is not limited to ordinary space, time, or ego boundaries. The sense of identity encompasses the totality of the universe. Separations and distinctions no longer exist, and the individual develops the perspective that everything, including oneself, is one with all. This expansion of one's identity from a separate and distinct ego to inclusion of an interconnected web of existence is known as ego disidentification. From this perspective, ordinary life is infused with a sense of the sacred (Robbins, Canda, & Chatterjee, 1998). Heightened empathy, compassion, and moral standards naturally arise as the individual experiences a profound connection with others (Canda & Furman, 1999; Dass & Gorman, 1985).

In addition, transpersonal experiences become more common in the transegoic stage. Grof (1988) developed a typology of clinically observed transpersonal experiences, which may include meditative states or altered states of consciousness, extrasensory perception, out of body experiences, and mystical or psychedelic experiences, and others in which the individual's awareness moves beyond space, time, and ego boundaries (Wilber, 1993). This theory views transpersonal experiences as crucial to the fulfillment of individuals at this level. Transpersonal theory focuses on a theoretical understanding of these experiences, the spiritual development process, and practice techniques that promote transpersonal awareness, healing, and transformation (Grof, 1988; Robbins, Canda, & Chatterjee, 1998).

Grof and Grof (1989) discussed the possibility of a spiritual emergency resulting from spiritual awakening. This may include a growing sense of dissatisfaction with the status quo and a sense that something is missing from life, factors which lead to depression. The individual may begin to inquire into the origin and purpose of life, and the meaning of suffering. A new value system may arise. Light, joy, energy, and visions may flood the person. If this transition into the transegoic stage occurs too quickly, the individual may have difficulty coping with it. Conventional psychology does not provide much support or explanation of these experiences other than labeling them as psychopathological. Without a positive cultural explanation of the source of these experiences, the individual may not understand them as a sign of spiritual development, and may instead interpret them as mental illness.

Transpersonal theorists generally agree that relatively few people achieve the transegoic stage of consciousness (Canda & Furman, 1999). Cultural factors may inhibit spiritual development, such as lack of access to resources which enhance growth, social and institutional structures which foster a sense of alienation and meaninglessness, social pressure toward egoism, and a world view which values materialism and a positivistic scientific method that considers as imaginary any experience beyond the five senses (Canda & Furman, 1999). This view particularly seems applicable to western society which places great value on individuality and personal control over the environment.

This author defines spirituality as a two-dimensional construct, including transcendence in terms of philosophy of life, and transcendence in terms of a sense of connection. Although a variety of definitions exists in current social work literature, reflecting both the wholeness of humanity and a component of one's experience (Carroll, 1998), often one or both of these dimensions are reflected in the definition. Canda (1990) defined spirituality as "the person's search for a sense of meaning and morally fulfilling relationships between oneself, other people, the encompassing universe, and the ontological ground of existence" (p. 13). Joseph (1987) defined spirituality as "the underlying dimension of consciousness which strives for meaning, union with the universe, and with all things; it extends to the experience of the transcendent or a power beyond us" (p. 14). In this author's understanding, both of these definitions may be interpreted to include a philosophical dimension involving purpose or meaning in life, as well as a sense of connection or union with others, the universe, and the transcendent.

The first dimension, transcendence in terms of philosophy of life, is cognitive in nature, and has to do with perspectives, values and belief systems about cosmology, the purpose of life, the nature of the universe, and one's place in it. Both religious and non-religious beliefs fit into this dimension. Philosophy of life becomes transcendent when it is focused on the welfare of all rather than one's own self-interest.

The second dimension, transcendence in terms of a sense of connection, is transrational and has to do with direct spiritual experience. This dimension may be described as a feeling of unity with the totality of the universe, a sense of oneness with God, others, nature, etc., communication with the spiritual dimension, peace of mind, a sense of compassion, or a sense of awareness of one's higher or spiritual self.

In the author's view, the dimensions influence each other, but are distinct. For example, an individual may hold a highly developed philosophy of life without undergoing direct spiritual experience. The philosophy may lead the person to conduct spiritual practice, which may then lead to transpersonal experience. A transpersonal experience will then most likely cause the individual to develop and revise his/her philosophy of life. Impacts of entry into the transegoic stage can be seen in both dimensions of spirituality, as will be discussed below.

The author has developed a taxonomy of major spiritual issues in terminal illness, which correspond with the two dimensions of spirituality. Meaning of life and suffering, unfinished business, and belief system correspond with the philosophy of life dimension. Major issues within the sense of connection dimension of spirituality include relationship with the Ultimate, isolation, and transpersonal experiences. These issues, along with a survey of hospice professionals which assesses the validity of the taxonomy of issues, are discussed in more detail elsewhere (Reese, 1999).

Spiritual Growth in Death and Dying

Evidence exists that confrontation with mortality spurs a period of spiritual growth in terminally ill patients (Herth, 1990; Peterson & Greil, 1990; Reed, 1987), their loved ones (Easley, 1987), and even in staff who work with them (Derezotes & Evans, 1995; Millison, 1988; Millison & Dudley, 1990). It may be difficult to test the relationships between spirituality and other variables in a sample of terminally ill patients due to the extremely high scores resulting from conventional spirituality scales (Reese, 1995-96). Furthermore, several studies have found consistent evidence that many terminally ill patients (Gibbs & Achterberg-Lawlis, 1978; Pflaum & Kelley, 1986; Reese, 1999) and their bereaved spouses (Simon-Buller, Christopherson, & Jones, 1988-89) report transpersonal experiences.

Gibbs and Achterberg-Lawlis (1978) reported that half of their sample of hospitalized terminally ill patients volunteered visions of God or other religious figures or deceased family members. These experiences were comforting, and the patients expressed relief in being able to discuss them without fear of rejection. Pflaum and Kelley (1986) found five commonly recurring themes in the experience of dying patients–(a) being in the presence of the dead, (b) preparing to travel or change, (c) seeing a place, (d) choosing when to die, and (e) knowing the time of death.

Reese (1999) conducted a survey of 66 terminally ill home hospice patients in Maryland and asked the question: "We have found that hospice patients often have spiritual experiences. Have you had any experiences that you would say are spiritual?" Nine patients declined to answer this question, some stating, "I don't want to talk about it." Of the remaining 57 patients, 44% responded in the affirmative. Their responses most often described near death experiences, in which deceased loved ones appeared to them, usually spouses or family members, although only one patient related the commonly described near death experience in which he traveled through a tunnel with a light at the end. The experiences might include a vision of a deceased spouse or family member coming to escort the patient, sometimes saying, "Come on," or telling the patient everything was going to be all right.

Three patients saw religious figures (Jesus or angels). One patient and his wife both saw a ray of light come through the yard and into the window, entering the patient's heart. One patient had an experience with precognition, in which he had a vision of his niece talking to his brother, just before the actual event which mirrored the vision. Only one patient described an experience, concerning clairvoyance, from his earlier life rather than during the dying process. An example summarized below, based on the words of the respondent, may help to clarify the nature of the author's data:

> The patient died of a heart attack, and went through a black tunnel with a tiny light at the end. He saw Jesus Christ in the tunnel, handing him a note. The patient had not lived a very moral life, and was afraid to look, because he was afraid the note would say he was going to hell. He finally looked at the note, which said, "I will show you the way." The note was signed, "Jesus Christ." At this point, the patient spontaneously resuscitated, and was filled with the holy spirit. The bed was shaking, the patient was shouting, the patient was saved and born again after that day. The Lord gave him scriptures he should read in church. He was a different person, he prayed for everybody. He saw Jesus at the foot of the bed again that night, and knew everything would be O.K. He kept saying to his wife, "Can't you see him?"

The above case description may be interpreted to indicate that terminal illness inspires a period of spiritual growth, with accompanying transpersonal experiences. According to Wilber (1995, 1996), transpersonal experiences occur within the highest stages of transpersonal development. There is a change in focus from concerns of the separate ego to a profound sense of connection with others (Canda & Furman, 1999). In this example, evidence of transpersonal growth can be seen in both dimensions of spirituality. Within the philosophy of life dimension, a change can be seen from concerns of the separate ego to a new life purpose and belief system. While before the transpersonal experience the patient had "not lived a very moral life," after the experience he attended church and read scriptures; he was "a different person." A change can also be seen within the sense of connection dimension–beginning with a lack of concern for others (not living a very moral life), the patient now "prayed for everybody." He also had frequent direct spiritual experiences, receiving guidance from "the Lord."

Consistent with this evidence about transpersonal growth in terminal illness, social workers report the importance of spirituality to terminally ill patients and their families (Derezotes & Evans, 1995; Reese & Brown, 1997).

HIV+ women report that spirituality is their most important way of coping with their illness (Reese & Kaplan, 1999), and research indicates that spirituality does impact client outcomes. Previous research by this author (Reese, 1995-96) clarifies its place in a model of variables. Specifically, spirituality reduces death anxiety and increases social support. The following discussion will use transpersonal theory to explain these relationships.

When faced with a terminal prognosis, an individual may become aware of his/her true nature separate from ego, identity, or role in society, facilitating transition into a transegoic perspective. A factor of death anxiety is fear of personal extinction (Conte, Weiner, & Plutchik, 1982), thus it makes sense that disidentification with the ego which occurs in the transegoic stage may reduce death anxiety (Smith, 1995). Development of a personal death perspective (Smith, 1995) has implications for the philosophical, cognitive dimension of spirituality. Thus, clients may benefit if social workers address major issues in this dimension.

As mentioned earlier, transpersonal theory also has implications for the nature of social relationships. As an individual experiences deep connection with others in the transegoic stage, compassion (Dass & Gorman, 1985) and heightened empathy (Canda & Furman, 1999) naturally arise. Personal gain ceases to be a prime objective; relationships are characterized by concern about the welfare of all. It is reasonable to expect that conflicts and competition would be reduced and relationships would improve. Thus, transpersonal theory helps to explain the impact of spirituality on social support. Entry into the transegoic stage with its perspective of oneness has implications for the sense of connection dimension of spirituality; thus, it is beneficial for social workers to address this dimension in practice as well.

Current Social Work Practice

Hospice philosophy and Medicare policy emphasize holistic care which includes attention to spiritual needs, and social workers, as part of the hospice team, are expected to address all aspects of holistic care, including spirituality (Dudley, Smith, & Millison, 1994; Millison & Dudley, 1992). Some studies indicate that social workers often address spirituality in practice with terminally ill patients (Derezotes, 1995; Reese & Brown, 1997, Russel, 2000), but Russel (2000) found that medical social workers address spirituality less often than mental health social workers. Evidence exists that spiritual assessment in hospice is conducted by social workers in a minority of cases, is not incorporated into the psychosocial treatment plan, and focuses mainly on religion and clergy involvement with the patient (Dudley et al., 1994). Several case studies have described successful social work intervention addressing spirituality

(Early, 1998; Reese, 1999; Smith, 1995; York, 1987), but few evaluation studies exist. Although some excellent practice models have been developed (i.e., Smith, 1995), the development of a theoretical base for social work interventions with spirituality is in its infancy.

Despite the inclusion of spirituality in the latest Council on Social Work Education curriculum guidelines (Council on Social Work Education Commission on Accreditation, 1995), little attention has been paid to spirituality in social work education (Derezotes, 1995; Russel, 1998; Sheridan, Bullis, Adcock, Berlin, & Miller, 1992). A recent survey by Quattlebaum and Cascio (1999) revealed that among graduate social work programs in the United States, only 27 social work programs offer courses on spirituality.

In summary, social workers address spirituality with terminally ill patients, but are unlikely to conduct a spiritual assessment and are likely to have little training in this area and to have produced few or no evaluation studies of the effectiveness of their spiritual interventions. In addition, few practice models exist; thus the interventions being used may lack a theoretical orientation. The inadequacy of training, lack of demonstration of effectiveness, and the lack of models for practice indicates a need for further work in this area. This article addresses this need by presenting a theoretical base and related techniques for social work intervention with spirituality in terminal illness, and providing results of a national survey documenting interventions and their impact on hospice outcomes.

NATIONAL HOSPICE SOCIAL WORK SURVEY

This article will report only partial results of the full study, which are relevant to hospice social work practice addressing spirituality.

Methodology

For the study as a whole, questionnaires were mailed to a stratified random sample of the National Hospice Organization membership. The original sample consisted of 350 hospices, with 75 hospices responding, for a response rate of 20%. Within each hospice, the director and the social worker each completed a questionnaire, and the social worker assigned to the case completed a chart review form for each of the most recently discharged cases. The questionnaires and forms provided quantitative as well as qualitative data. For data analysis purposes, only hospices which provided the social work questionnaire and all five cases were included in the analysis; thus, the final sample size used for this analysis was 65 hospices and social workers and 325 patients. According to accepted qualitative methodology, feedback was sought from these participants about the credibility and meaning of the results.

Information was collected about social work services and hospice outcomes. Measures were selected from the literature or developed by the researchers with input from expert social workers in the field. Hospice outcome variables relevant to these results include: family functioning, measured by the McMaster Family Assessment Device (Epstein, Baldwin, & Bishop, 1983); severity of case, measured by a scale developed from the Social Work Acuity Scale for Hospice (Runnion, undated); and bereavement risk, measured by the Bereavement Risk Index (Parkes & Weiss, 1983). Reliability for these scales was tested using Cronbach's alpha, with alpha equaling .87 for the McMaster Family Assessment Device, .70 for the revised Social Work Acuity Scale, and .31 for the Bereavement Risk Index.

Results

The findings indicate that a total of 72.7% of the social workers held a negative view of the attention paid to spirituality in their social work education programs, with 29.8% viewing their training as inadequate, and 42.9% as very much inadequate. MSWs were significantly less likely than BSWs to rate the attention to spirituality as adequate (t = 3,186, df = 196, Sig. = .002). New graduates indicated more adequate attention to spirituality than more experienced social workers (correlation between months of experience since degree and adequacy of attention to spirituality, r = −.246, p = .001).

Despite this lack of training, 58% of social workers said they addressed spirituality with their interdisciplinary teams. This data was collected by a qualitative question on the social work questionnaire asking respondents to circle spirituality if they had provided input to their teams in this area, and to give an example of such input. This qualitative data, analyzed by the constant comparative method, provided in-depth information about the interventions provided. These interventions are reported in Table 1. Three percent of the social workers had an official role in addressing spirituality in the hospice–for example, were responsible for conducting the spiritual assessment. Six percent, however, stated they only address spirituality if a chaplain is unavailable.

The chart review forms also provided qualitative data about social work interventions with spirituality in individual patient cases. Data analysis revealed that the issues addressed were generally consistent with the author's taxonomy of major spiritual issues. Interventions addressing major spiritual issues in counseling were self-reported on the social work questionnaire by 23% of the social workers. In contrast to this figure, however, qualitative analysis of the

TABLE 1. Self-Report of Spiritual Topics Addressed by Social Workers with Team

% of social workers (n = 65)	Topic addressed
3%	Had official role in addressing spirituality in the hospice, i.e., responsible for the spiritual assessment
6%	Only addressed spirituality if a chaplain is unavailable
23%	Provided counseling regarding spiritual issues with patients and families
22%	Advocated with the team to honor spiritual diversity
12%	Obtained spiritual support for patients and families
8%	Advocated for spiritual care for the team
6%	Identified the spiritual orientation and beliefs of the patient and family
6%	Educated the team regarding distinction between spirituality and religion
6%	Identified spiritual issues concerning the patient and family
3%	Identified spiritual supports outside hospice
2%	Identified spiritual interventions that could be used with patient and family
1%	Attended the memorial service held by the hospice for patients
5%	Reported that they address spirituality with the team, but did not specify how

chart review form data indicates that 62% of the social workers actually addressed spiritual issues in counseling sessions with clients.

A breakdown of the issues addressed is shown in Table 2. The table provides the percent of social workers reporting that in general they have addressed a specific spiritual issue in counseling with clients at some point during their practice at the hospice, the percent of social workers actually addressing a spiritual issue at some point according to the chart review information, and the percent of cases in which each issue was addressed according to the chart review. Although many more social workers than reported were actually addressing spirituality at some point with clients, the actual percentage of cases receiving such interventions is low.

Some examples of interventions with meaning of life and suffering include reminiscing and life review and exploring opportunities for the patient to contribute to research regarding his or her illness. Interventions with unfinished business included work on forgiveness, discussion of use of remaining time, and coordinating an out of state trip for the patient and significant other. Social workers addressed client belief systems by exploring beliefs about the afterlife

TABLE 2. Major Spiritual Issues Addressed, by Self-Report and Chart Review

	% of social workers addressing issue (n = 65)		
Major spiritual issue	By Self-report	According to chart review	% of cases in which issue was addressed - according to chart review (n = 325)
Meaning of life and suffering	5%	43%	13%
Unfinished business	0%	12%	3.3%
Belief system	2%	40%	12.7%
Relationship with the Ultimate	0%	0%	0%
Isolation	2%	26%	5.5%
Transpersonal experiences	5%	6%	1.8%

Note: Social workers may have addressed more than one issue, and more than one issue may have been addressed in each case.

and discussing the reasons for the patient's death anxiety. Relationship with the Ultimate was not addressed by this sample, although it was the most frequently addressed issue according to a chart review conducted in an Illinois hospice (Reese & Brown, 1997). Interventions with isolation included validating the patient's need to talk openly about the illness and death, requesting that the children contact the patient, and helping the patient and family say goodbye to the patient, let go, and give permission for the patient to die. Interventions with transpersonal experiences included discussion of near death experiences, validation of the family's prayer for a miracle, validation of the therapeutic use of prayer, encouraging the use of prayer, and praying at the bedside with the patient and caregiver. Table 3 summarizes interventions used by this sample with each issue.

Correlation results clarified hospice characteristics which enabled social workers to address spirituality more frequently. Social work visits to patients are unfortunately fairly infrequent in hospice, with the median number of contacts with a patient for this sample equaling 2. If a social worker had the opportunity to visit patients more frequently, however, the social worker addressed spirituality more often during the visit (total social work contacts/addressing unfinished business: $r = .12$, $p = .03$; total social work contacts/addressing meaning of life and suffering: $r = .11$, $p = .05$). This opportunity for more visits was likely due to a higher full-time equivalency of social workers in the hos-

TABLE 3. Summary of Interventions Used by Sample to Address Each Major Spiritual Issue

MAJOR ISSUES: Philosophy of life dimension	INTERVENTIONS USED
Meaning of life and suffering	Reminiscing Life review Discussing meaning of life Discussing meaning of decline/death Family discussion of value of patient's life
Unfinished business	Completion of life tasks Explored research opportunities Worked on forgiveness Discussion of use of remaining time Coordinated out-of-state trip
Belief system	

MAJOR ISSUES: Sense of connection dimension	
Relationship with the Ultimate	No interventions documented
Isolation	Discussed importance of talking openly Discussed importance of relationships Helped patient and caregiver to express feelings Requested children contact patient
Transpersonal experiences	Validation of family's beliefs in a miracle Validation of caregiver's prayer for a miracle Validation of use of prayer Discussion of near death experiences Prayed at bedside with patient and caregiver

pice (fulltime social work equivalent/social worker obtaining spiritual support in the case: $r = .20$, $p = .002$) and higher revenues set aside to provide social work services in the hospice (higher social work costs/social worker obtaining spiritual support in the case: $r = .16$, $p = .03$).

Correlation testing also revealed some characteristics of clients which may predict whether social workers address spirituality in the case. The literature indicates that lower income clients, often from ethnic or racial minorities, as a result of discrimination, may rely on spirituality in times of crisis more than the dominant culture (Reese, Ahern, Nair, O'Faire, & Warren, 1999). Results of this study show that social workers are more likely to address the belief system with lower income clients (client income/social worker addressing belief system: $r = .18$, $p = .01$). In addition, the spirituality of the significant other of the patient predicts how often the social worker addresses transpersonal experiences in the case ($r = .14$, $p = .032$).

Finally, impact of social work intervention with spirituality on patient outcomes was assessed with bivariate correlational procedures. The family functioning score was predicted by the total number of spiritual issues addressed by the social worker in the case ($r = .16$, $p = .01$), and by the number of referrals for chaplain visits ($r = .17$, $p = .004$). A result that was close to significance, and of particular interest here, was that the degree to which the social worker addressed transpersonal issues predicted the severity of the case ($r = -.11$, $p = .08$).

DISCUSSION

Limitations of the Study

Limitations of the study must be kept in mind when interpreting results.

1. The poor response rate (20%) may limit generalizability of findings, although sample patient demographics parallel national statistics (National Hospice Organization, 1999).
2. The poor reliability for the Bereavement Risk Scale limits confidence in the findings; further research is needed regarding this variable.
3. Internal validity is an issue, as with all survey studies. It was not possible to document all other factors influencing variable relationships; one concern is that other professions on the team may have been addressing spirituality with the clients, thus making it difficult to identify the separate effects of social work intervention. One should note, though, that previous research indicates chaplains visit less frequently than social workers, and that social workers address spirituality more frequently than nurses (Reese, 1995-96; Reese & Brown, 1997).
4. Definition of spirituality was a factor influencing the results. If we had defined spirituality for the social workers, the self-report of interventions may have been different. However, we do have the objective chart review data. The fact that we did not define spirituality for participants allows us to observe the disparity between their self-report and the chart review, which provides interesting information about the inability to define spirituality and identify spiritual issues. Social workers may be unaware of the distinction between spirituality and religion, but they should be aware of hospice thinking regarding major issues faced by patients and families. They may be unable to identify some of them as spiritual issues, but they should be addressing them with most if not all clients.
5. Finally, the author recognizes a possible bias in analyzing qualitative results; her conclusions indicate that the spiritual issues addressed by social workers in the sample correspond with her taxonomy of major

spiritual issues. This bias was addressed to an extent by assigning the qualitative analysis to a research assistant.

Participant Feedback

In order to provide triangulation of the data, the author's conclusions were forwarded to the participants for feedback. Two questions (summarized here) were included in the letter:

1. How would you explain the result that more social workers addressed spiritual issues than reported it? Are social workers defining spirituality differently than the author is, or having difficulty identifying spiritual issues due to lack of training?
2. How would you explain the result that the majority of cases were not receiving social work intervention with spirituality? Did the small number of visits limit the social work intervention to assessment rather than extensive counseling, or do social workers believe it is inappropriate to address spirituality? Or do they find it difficult to address spirituality due to lack of training?

Six participants responded to the request for feedback. Their comments were analyzed again by the constant comparative method, and two major themes emerged, as discussed below:

1. Social work education. A number of the factors explaining the results of the study could be addressed through social work education:
   (a) *Definition of spirituality.* Although a participant stated agreement with the author's definition, social workers may be confusing spirituality with religion, or otherwise defining spirituality in a different way.
   (b) *Lack of training.* Participants reported an absence of discussion of spirituality in their social work education also and reported that inclusion of both content on end of life care and spirituality would be helpful. One participant felt qualified to address spirituality despite the lack of training, due to personal and professional experience. Participants related plans to address these issues. One hospice is beginning discussions with local colleges and universities regarding the need for training. One hospice made the point that their budget does not allow for a full-time chaplain; thus they will be utilizing their volunteer clergy in training the staff to be more comfortable with addressing spiritual issues.
   (c) *Not documenting spiritual intervention.* Many social workers probably do not document addressing spiritual concerns.

(d) *Values of social workers.* Although participants expressed that they believe it is appropriate for social workers to address spirituality, one participant stated that it's not until one gets into hospice that a social worker finds out it's O.K., and that this belief may be unique to hospice.

(e) *Social worker's personal issues.* It may be difficult emotionally for social workers to address spirituality because it touches one's own fears. A participant also expressed, however, that the emotional impact of hospice work is what gives it its meaning.

(f) *Clinical issues.* Many clients may be unwilling to talk about their beliefs, or may be actively dying and unable to talk with the social worker.

2. *Hospice policy.* A number of factors affecting social work intervention with spirituality are influenced by hospice policy.

(a) *The hospice budget, along with short length of stay* by patients, may only allow for a low number of social work visits and a lack of time with clients in the hospice, limiting social work services to assessment rather than counseling. Also the budget may not include paid chaplain services; full-time chaplains may be more able to train the team to address spiritual issues.

(b) *Interdisciplinary relationships.* Although hospice philosophy holds that all members of the team should address spirituality, sometimes spirituality is considered the chaplain's domain. Social workers may do the initial spiritual assessment, but not intervention with spiritual issues. There may be turf issues between chaplains and social workers or chaplains may define spirituality differently from social workers, or social workers may feel that the chaplains are well qualified to address such issues and leave this responsibility up to them.

IMPLICATIONS FOR PRACTICE

These results of the National Hospice Social Work Survey (NHSWS) indicate that although hospice social workers are addressing spirituality, they are not trained to do so and are unable to identify a client concern as a spiritual issue. This is consistent with a participant's comment in a study by Canda (1988a) that social workers are involved in deeply spiritual activity, but often lack awareness of it. Similarly, Graham, Kaiser, and Garrett (1998) argue that the core of the helping relationship is spiritual, but that social workers do not recognize and name spiritual questions as such. It will be impossible to conduct an adequate spiritual assessment unless the social worker is able to identify and elicit discussion of major spiritual issues.

This situation raises ethical questions, such as whether the social workers are imposing their own belief systems on clients, and whether there is a probable failure to practice within the accepted social work body of knowledge regarding spirituality in practice. Although the majority of social workers in the NHSWS were addressing spirituality at some point with some client, spirituality was still not addressed in the vast majority of cases. Almost half of social workers failed to address spirituality with their teams, and 29% failed to address it with clients at all. Relationship with the Ultimate was not addressed, despite being the most frequently addressed issue in one hospice in Illinois (Reese & Brown, 1997), and transpersonal experiences were rarely addressed with clients despite evidence that many terminally ill patients may be having these experiences (Gibbs & Achterberg-Lawlis, 1978; Pflaum & Kelley, 1986; Reese, 1999). Further development of models of practice is needed, and publication of models which are being used in practice but have not been disseminated to the profession as a whole. Further research is needed, subsequently, to test these practice models for effectiveness.

Regardless of the lack of training and lack of models for practice, the lack of deliberate and explicit effort to address spirituality, and the low frequency of addressing it, results surprisingly still show an impact on client outcomes from social work intervention with spiritual concerns. One would expect even better client outcomes with specific training in this area. Training is needed which develops skills in defining spirituality, identifying issues, and the use of intervention techniques; Canda (1991) suggests that conventional and transpersonal theories be placed together in the curriculum to provide breadth and diversity of perspectives. Social work education should address the importance of spirituality to low income and diverse populations. Qualitative feedback from study respondents suggests that social work education could also address values about whether social workers should address spirituality, personal issues of the social worker which inhibit intervention in this area, clinical issues for clients which pose barriers, and proper documentation of spiritual interventions in patient charts.

A number of hospice policy issues also need to be addressed in order to permit adequate spiritual care. Results show that budgeting for increased social work and chaplain services increases intervention with spiritual issues. Turf issues between social workers and chaplains need to be resolved, perhaps by interdisciplinary training in this area. Finally, the short length of stay in hospice needs to be addressed at a programmatic and national level; Medicare regulations need to be reviewed for barriers to referral, and transitional programs including both palliative care and hospice need to be developed.

Use of Transpersonal Theory

Results of the National Hospice Social Work Survey indicate that hospice social workers have a lack of training for addressing spirituality. Despite the

lack of training and the lack of existing models for practice in this area, the issues addressed were generally consistent with the author's taxonomy of major
spiritual issues, and the interventions provided had a significant impact on client outcomes. Interventions used by the sample are summarized in Table 3.
The following discussion addresses the need for models of practice, and provides a general theoretical background. It suggests general interventions for
promoting transition into the transegoic stage of consciousness and techniques
for helping clients resolve each major spiritual issue. The techniques described
clarify techniques listed in Table 3, as well as providing additional approaches
for social work intervention.

The above theoretical discussion and research results indicate that interventions which foster a transpersonal perspective can be very helpful to clients,
specifically in reducing death anxiety and increasing social support. The two
dimensions of spirituality, which represent respectively an intellectual perspective and an experiential awareness, call for therapeutic techniques addressing both levels–in other words, both discussions on a rational level and
experiential exercises. Rational discussions can help clients to develop new
perspectives, and the use of guided imagery and symbolism can facilitate
changes beyond the rational level, with a revised intellectual perspective resulting from these experiences as well.

Experiential techniques can be quite powerful, effecting dramatic changes
and major therapeutic breakthroughs over a short period of time. Due to the
possible intensity of the experience, however, many authors note cautions
when using experiential techniques. Canda and Furman (1999) advise social
workers not to "try out" new techniques on clients which they have never used
before. The social worker should be competent in the approach, through specific
training if possible, and definitely through significant personal experience with
the technique. In addition, social workers should exercise caution if the client is
fragile psychologically or physically, and gear the techniques accordingly.
Adults should have a well-established ego before it is safe to transcend it. In particular, psychotic patients may have difficulty in practicing techniques which
foster an altered state of consciousness. If the technique requires a physical capacity that the client doesn't have (for example, a breathing technique when the
client is using oxygen and has difficulty breathing) a more appropriate technique
should be chosen for that client. But often simple exercises are helpful in reducing the symptoms of mental or physical disorders (Canda & Furman, 1999).

Finally, interventions to address spirituality should only be used with the client's permission and only after explaining the purpose of the technique. Assess-
ments should gather information about the client's belief system, and contracting
should determine the issues the client is interested in exploring. Interventions
should reflect the client's belief system and the agreed upon treatment plan.

The following suggests interventions for social work practice addressing spirituality in hospice. Many of the techniques have effects on more than one major spiritual issue, and all promote transition into the transegoic stage of consciousness.

General Techniques

A number of techniques generally promote transition into the transegoic stage, without specifically addressing a major spiritual issue. First, teaching traditional meditation practice and practicing with the client can be very valuable in promoting spiritual growth (Bullis, 1996; Grof & Grof, 1989) as well as stress relief. Meditation can take many forms; Canda and Furman (1999) describe basic meditation techniques which include: (a) *Paying attention*–helps patients to develop mindfulness and awareness of the true essence of being (for example, savor a shower, treasure each moment with a loved one, realize that each moment is precious); (b) *Intentional breathing*–relieves stress, helps further to pay attention. One can add a mantra, either religious, or one's own thought (for example, "Peace" on the inbreath, "For all" on the outbreath). In addition, Bullis (1996) has developed an approach to meditation which includes relaxation, visualization, affirmation, confirmation, appreciation, and conclusion.

Assagioli (1977) developed the Exercise of the Blossoming of the Rose to promote transpersonal development. The client visualizes the development of a rose from a bud, which symbolizes his/her own spiritual development. The visualization involves looking at a rosebush, visualizing one stem with leaves and a rosebud. The bud begins to separate very slowly, until a fully open rose is visualized. Visualize smelling the perfume, expanding the vision to include the whole rosebush. Imagine the life force that arises from the roots to the flower and that originates the process of opening. Identify with the rose–symbolically we are this rose–the same life that animates the universe and has created the miracle of the rose is producing in us a like, even greater miracle–the awakening and development of our spiritual being and that which radiates from it. This is a visualization technique that can be used with hospice patients even if weak and bedridden. It can promote awareness of spiritual wellness, even in the presence of severe physical debility.

Other techniques which foster transition into the transegoic stage include movement meditation, group chanting, giving full expression to one's emotions through the use of music, working with dreams, drawing and painting, keeping a journal, Jungian active imagination, Fritz Perls' gestalt practice, acupuncture, and Grof's Holotropic Breathwork (Grof & Grof, 1989).

Meaning of Life and Suffering

Reminiscing or life review is often used to help clients see crisis as an opportunity for transpersonal growth (Robbins et al., 1998), and to discover their transpersonal missions (Smith & Gray, 1995). A powerful approach to life review is Bullis's (1996) spiritual genogram exercise, which charts a client's spiritual family tree. The client draws his/her conceptualization of spiritual ancestors, including significant books, experiences, lectures, events, relatives, and friends, which have shaped his/her spiritual orientation or outlook. The genogram may be in the form of a time line, which represents the map of the client's life. After completion of the genogram, the client can see more clearly the impact that peak events, nadir experiences, and plateau experiences (Maslow, 1970) have had on his/her transpersonal development. Evidence of the growth resulting from adversity helps the client to accept past trauma, find meaning in suffering, and develop a belief system which includes a personal death perspective. A hospice patient is often able to perceive positive outcomes resulting from negative past events, and even from terminality (for example, in the resolution of conflicts with others, reconnection with their family, etc). This exercise could help a client to answer the common question, "Why would God do this to me?" In developing an individual answer to this question, a client develops a personal death perspective, which promotes transpersonal growth in the philosophy of life dimension of spirituality.

Other ways of finding meaning include meditation (Canda, 1988b), journaling (Smith, 1993), discussion of dreams and drawings (Early, 1998), and life review. The social worker should be open to the possibility that some clients will be unable to engage in direct reflection about death and dying. In this case, the worker can simply offer his/her presence (Owen-Still, 1985).

Unfinished Business

As an individual begins to develop a transpersonal perspective, reconciliation with events or other people may be needed. Several authors suggest planning for the use of remaining time, with the aim of completing unfinished business (Early, 1998; Peay, 1997; Reese, 1999). Unfinished business may include resolution of prior grief (Smith & Gray, 1995), accomplishing final goals, or resolving concerns regarding sin, guilt, and the need for forgiveness of self and others (Canda & Furman, 1999; Loewenberg, 1988; Reese, 1999). A case example is a hospice patient who had been living with his partner for a number of years, and according to his belief system, he felt he should make her "an honest woman" by marrying her. The hospice chaplain was called to the bedside to perform the ceremony, helping the patient to conclude unfinished business and to die in peace.

Reconciliation with estranged loved ones becomes quite important to some patients on their death beds, thus social work skills in this area are needed. Worthington and DiBlasio (1990) outline techniques for promoting mutual forgiveness within troubled relationships, including owning one's hurtful actions, eschewing future hurtfulness, forgiving the partner for past hurts, perhaps atonement for hurting the partner, and sacrifice for each partner.

Another social work responsibility is helping patients to resolve feelings of guilt due to past actions. For example, one hospice patient struggled with guilt over killing enemy soldiers during a war. In another example, a Catholic patient agonized with a past abortion, which she viewed as sin, and questioned whether God had stricken her with cancer as a punishment.

In some cases, religious ritual may help the client to resolve guilt; if the client is interested, the social worker should make a referral to the appropriate religious leader. Referral to a clergy member may allow resolution of issues falling under the responsibility of the church, such as marriage, reconciliation of the client with his church, or resolution of issues specific to religious beliefs (Reese, 1999). In the case of the Catholic patient mentioned above, a referral was made to the priest on the hospice team, who helped her to resolve her sin and guilt through her own belief system.

Loewenberg (1988) outlines assessment of whether there is an objective reason for the guilt or whether it is based on imagined transgressions. If the guilt is real, he suggests helping the client to transform guilt-producing behavior into a more moral and satisfying behavior. Acceptance of the individual, while not condoning unethical behaviors, can be an important support in resolving this issue. Loewenberg also suggests helping the client refocus on strengths. Alternatively, if the guilt is not based on actual misdeeds, the social worker should help the client to understand the irrational basis for his feelings (Loewenberg, 1988). The determination of whether or not an act is unethical should be based on the client's own belief system and not the worker's beliefs.

Swett (personal communication, 1990) has developed a powerful guided imagery technique for assisting clients in forgiving past hurts, even in situations where face-to-face contact between the client and the one he/she needs to forgive is impossible. In this exercise, the client imagines an umbilical cord connecting him/her to the person he/she needs to forgive. The client imagines a filter on this connection so that only positive energy, not negative, may flow through. Next the client imagines positive spiritual energy flowing through him/herself, through the umbilical cord, and through the other person, so that all are washed clean of negative energy. If necessary, the connection may be cut altogether and the other person allowed to go his/her own way.

If clients have strong regrets over investing their lives in secular pursuits, one last noble act, such as donating an organ, changing one negative pattern, or making a donation, may help to alleviate these regrets (Peay, 1997). Peay describes a dying woman who was bitter over life events and was helped by a hospice priest to dedicate her dying as a way to alleviate the suffering of a young bereaved mother. The patient was transformed, her whole being was "infused with radiant love," and her thoughts were focused on praying for and helping the young mother (Peay, 1997).

Early (1998) describes asking a dying adolescent if there were things he would like to do before he died, and helping the client to address these issues with his family. Finally, Canda and Furman (1999) discuss the healing impact that rituals may have, whether religious or developed to symbolize the issue at hand, in resolving the emotional impact of traumatic experiences.

Belief System

Working on death anxiety may entail development of a belief system, and Peay (1997) and Bullis (1996) suggest deliberately bringing up the question of the client's beliefs. Peay suggests reading passages and examining various belief systems on the topic. Smith (1993) suggests using a spiritual journal in which the client writes down any thoughts or feelings about God, the afterlife, religion, or spirituality.

Several models, including Assagioli's psychosynthesis (1977), specifically focus on helping the client to develop a transpersonal belief system. The exercise in disidentification (Assagioli) asks the client to affirm with conviction and become aware of the facts that "I have a body, but I am not my body. I have an emotional life, but I am not my emotions or my feelings. I have an intellect, but I am not that intellect. I am I, a center of pure consciousness." The "I" can observe and control these other aspects of the self. Through developing this perspective, the individual gains the ability to disidentify with these parts of the self and to become aware of the transpersonal essence of his/her being. This new perspective, then, helps to reduce death anxiety.

Assagioli (1977) developed an additional exercise asking the client to answer the question: "Who am I?" The client will usually reply from the perspective of his societal roles. After this reply, ask him again to respond to the same question. Each successive time, the client will respond with a deeper answer, more reflective of a transpersonal perspective on the nature of the self.

Smith's (1995) transegoic model also facilitates transpersonal development into the transegoic stage and includes the stages of normalization of death, faith in the existential self, ego disattachment, and self-transcendence. Another approach to helping the client disidentify with his/her ego and social roles includes visualizing letting go of roles that have defined the client (Peay, 1997).

Relationship with the Ultimate

Relationship with God was the most frequently addressed issue, regardless of profession, in a recent study of spiritual and psychosocial issues addressed with patients by hospice staff (Reese & Brown, 1997). Resolution of problems in this area can promote a sense of unity with all. A technique which can be used to promote a sense of connection to the Ultimate is the Spiritual Shower (Swett, undated) in which the client is asked to visualize white spiritual light in the form of a shower flowing over and through him/her, entering in through the top of the head and flowing out of the hands and feet. At first, the light washes out any darkness, areas of sickness, or negative energy or emotion. Then, the client is asked to visualize that the holes in the hands and feet are closed, and the light then fills the client, filling any empty spaces, and finally spilling out the pores of the body to fill an impenetrable bubble of light. Other approaches to this issue include discussions of worthiness to God (Early, 1998; Reese, 1999), work on developmental issues which affect the client's concept of God (Joseph, 1988), referral to a clergy member to discuss specific religious beliefs (Early, 1988), and art depicting one's conceptualization of God (Smith, 1993).

Isolation

A number of issues can interfere with the client's sense of connection and unity. One of the things social workers do best is to help restore close relationships and resolve conflicts with others. Useful approaches include helping clients and families explore ways to maintain intimacy, stressing the importance of sharing feelings as a way to cope, helping a family reassure the client that it is acceptable to talk to them about illness and death, and arranging meetings between clients and those with which they want to be reconciled. Hospice itself may serve as a cohesive community that promotes a sense of belonging for the client, and the relationship between the social worker and client can in itself lead to an increased awareness of one's commonality with the rest of humanity (Graham et al., 1998). Finally, Canda and Furman (1999) note the impact of mutually beneficial human-nature relationships in experiencing a profound sense of connection.

Transpersonal Experiences

Transpersonal experiences are common in the transegoic stage (Grof, 1988), and there is evidence that they occur frequently during death and dying (Gibbs & Achterberg-Lawlis, 1978; Pflaum & Kelley, 1986; Reese, 1999). Peay (1997) recommends asking clients directly if they have ever had a mystical experience of union with the universe. It may be helpful to tell the client about one's own transpersonal experiences, either to normalize the client's experiences or to encourage a client who has not had such experiences. For example, a hospice social worker known to this author tells his clients about his own near death experience, and reports that they find it a comfort.

In addition, hospice clients frequently bring up transpersonal experiences for discussion. It is important for the social worker to respond appropriately, with respect and without judgment or imposing one's own belief system. An example is a patient's son who related to this author that he believed his mother saw an angel at the foot of her bed shortly before death. It is important to distinguish between the psychosocial and spiritual dimensions (Graham et al., 1998; Robbins et al., 1998), and essential not to interpret the client's experience in a materialistic way (Grof & Grof, 1989). "To give only psychological or sociological answers to spiritual questions represents a failure to fully hear the client and be 'where the client is' " (Graham et al., 1998, p. 53). It is vital to help the family to accept and support the patient's experiences (Pflaum & Kelley, 1986). The social worker should educate the client on the normalcy and nature of transpersonal experiences during spiritual growth, including the commonly occurring experiences of both bliss and depression. The social worker should provide a positive context for the experiences, and assert that it is worth it to go through such experiences because of the outcome of transition into the transegoic stage (Grof & Grof, 1989). The social worker should help the client to understand the meaning and symbolism of their experiences and to resolve any issues symbolized by the experience (Pflaum & Kelley, 1986). Grof (1988) describes the role of the therapist in response to transpersonal experiences as supporting the experiential process with full trust in its healing nature, without trying to change it, even without full understanding of its meaning.

CONCLUSION

This article proposed that transition into the transegoic stage of development promotes a comfortable death for hospice patients due to reducing death anxiety and enhancing social support. Transpersonal theory can be used as a basis for assessment and practice models for social work intervention with this population.

A study was reported which indicates a lack of social work training in this area, an inability to define spirituality according to current social work literature, and an inability to identify major spiritual issues. Despite the lack of training and lack of explicit attempts to address spirituality, social work intervention with spiritual issues beneficially affected client outcomes. Interventions used by the sample were presented, and additional interventions were suggested to address each of six major spiritual issues. Suggestions were given for hospice policy change, including budgeting for psychosocial and spiritual care, and resolving interdisciplinary relationship issues between social workers and chaplains.

Areas that should be addressed by social work education include the definition of spirituality, identification of spiritual issues, models of practice that can be used to address these issues with terminally ill clients and families, diverse spiritual beliefs and values about honoring diversity, proper documentation of spiritual interventions, values about the importance of addressing spirituality, personal issues of social workers that inhibit them from addressing spirituality, and approaches to address client difficulty in discussing spiritual issues.

In the end, the people who are dying will teach us these lessons more often than we will teach them. The experience of dying propels many people into a transegoic perspective, which they pass on to their loved ones and the staff working with them.

> The most beautiful Americans I've been around are people who are almost dead. That is because they're not busy being lost in their identity–such as being rich, poor, fat, smart, needy, Buddhist, or the adult child of an alcoholic. Those things aren't too important when you're dying and you're whittled down to an essential level of being. Thus, to the extent that we can carry our identities a little more lightly before death, so much the better. That's what the dying teach the living. (Dale Borglum, quoted by Peay 1997, p. 11)

REFERENCES

Assagioli, R. (1977). *Psychosynthesis: A manual of principles and techniques.* New York: Penguin Books.

Bullis, R. (1996). *Spirituality in social work practice.* Washington, D.C.: Taylor & Francis.

Canda, E. (1988a). Conceptualizing spirituality for social work: Insights from diverse perspectives. *Social Thought, 14*(1), 30-46.

Canda, E. (1988b). Spirituality, religious diversity, and social work practice. *Social Casework, 69*(4), 238-247.

Canda, E. (1990). Afterword: Spirituality reexamined. *Spirituality and Social Work Communicator, 1*(1), 13-14.

Canda, E. (1991). East/West philosophical synthesis in transpersonal theory. *Journal of Sociology and Social Welfare, 18*(4), 137-152.

Canda, E., & Furman, L. (1999). *Spiritual diversity in social work practice: The heart of helping.* New York: The Free Press.

Carroll, M. (1998). Social work's conceptualization of spirituality. In E. Canda (Ed.), *Spirituality in social work: New directions* (pp. 1-13). New York: The Haworth Press, Inc.

Conte, H., Weiner, M., & Plutchik, R. (1982). Measuring death anxiety: Conceptual, psychometric, and factor-analytic aspects. *Journal of Personality and Social Psychology, 4*(4), 775-785.

Council on Social Work Education Commission on Accreditation. (1995). *Handbook of accreditation standards and procedures.* Alexandria, VA: Council on Social Work Education.

Dass, R., & Gorman, P. (1985). *How can I help? Stories and reflections on service.* New York: Knopf.

Derezotes, D. (1995). Spirituality and religiosity: Neglected factors in social work practice. *Arete, 20*(1), 1-15.

Derezotes, D., & Evans, K. (1995). Spirituality and religiosity in practice: In-depth interviews of social work practitioners. *Social Thought, 18*(1), 39-56.

Dudley, J., Smith, C., & Millison, M. (1994). Unfinished business: Assessing the spiritual needs of hospice clients. *Healing Ministry, (March/April),* 8-15.

Early, B. (1998). Between two worlds: The psychospiritual crisis of a dying adolescent. *Social Thought: Journal of Religion in the Social Services, 18*(2), 67-80.

Easley, E. (1987). The impact of traumatic events on religious faith: Implications for social work. *Dissertation Abstracts, 23*(3), No. 1050.

Epstein, N., Baldwin, L., & Bishop, S. (1983). The McMaster Family Assessment Device. *Journal of Marital and Family Therapy, 9,* 171-180.

Gibbs, H., & Achterberg-Lawlis, J. (1978). Spiritual values and death anxiety: Implications for counseling with terminal cancer patients. *Journal of Counseling Psychology, 25,* 563-569.

Graham, M., Kaiser, T., & Garrett, K. (1998). Naming the spiritual: The hidden dimension of helping. *Social Thought, 18*(4), 49-61.

Grof, S. (1988). *The adventure of self-discovery.* Albany, NY: State University of New York Press.

Grof, S., & Grof, C. (1989). *Spiritual emergency.* New York: Putnam.

Herth, K. (1990). Fostering hope in terminally ill people. *Journal of Advanced Nursing, 15*(11), 1250-1259.

Joseph, M. V. (1987). The religious and spiritual aspects of social work practice: A neglected dimension of social work. *Social Thought, 13*(1), 12-23.

Joseph, M. V. (1988). Religion and social work practice. *Social Casework, 69,* 443-452.

Loewenberg, F. (1988). *Religion and social work practice in contemporary American society.* New York: Columbia University Press.

Maslow, A. (1970). *Religion, values, and peak experiences.* New York: Viking.

Millison, M. (1988). Spirituality and the caregiver: Developing an underutilized facet of care. *The American Journal of Hospice Care, March/April,* 37-44.

Millison, M., & Dudley, J. (1990). The importance of spirituality in hospice work: A study of hospice professionals. *The Hospice Journal, 6*(3), 63-78.

Millison, M., & Dudley, J. (1992). Providing spiritual support: A job for all hospice professionals. *The Hospice Journal, 8*(4), 49-66.

National Hospice Organization. (1999). *NHO Hospice fact sheet.* Arlington, VA: Author.

Owen-Still, S. (1985). Spiritual caregiving: A philosophy for the volunteer-intensive hospice program. *The American Journal of Hospice Care, March/April,* 32-35.

Parkes, C. M., & Weiss, R. S. (1983). *Recovery from bereavement.* New York: Basic Books.

Peay, P. (1997, Sept./Oct.). A good death. *Common Boundary.* [On-line]. (Available: commonboundary.org)

Peterson, S., & Greil, A. (1990). Death experience and religion. *Omega, 21*(1), 75-82.

Pflaum, M., & Kelley, P. (1986). Understanding the final messages of the dying. *Nursing, 16*(60), 26-29.

Quattlebaum, A., & Cascio, T. (1999). *National survey findings: Design and implementation of coursework intersecting spirituality and practice.* Paper presented at the Annual Program Meeting of the Council on Social Work Education, San Francisco, CA.

Reed, P. (1987). Spirituality and wellbeing in terminally ill hospitalized adults. *Research in Nursing and Health, 10*(5), 335-44.

Reese, D. (formerly Ita, D.). (1995-96). Testing of a causal model: Acceptance of death in hospice patients. *Omega: Journal of Death and Dying, 32*(2), 81-92.

Reese, D. (1999). Spirituality conceptualized as purpose in life and sense of connection: Major issues and counseling approaches with terminal illness. *Healing Ministry, 6*(3), 101-108.

Reese, D., Ahern, R., Nair, S., O'Faire, J., & Warren, C. (1999). Hospice access and utilization by African Americans: Addressing cultural and institutional barriers through participatory action research. *Social Work, 44*(6), 549-559.

Reese, D., & Brown, D. (1997). Psychosocial and spiritual care in hospice: Differences between nursing, social work, and clergy. *The Hospice Journal, 12*(1), 29-41.

Reese, D., & Kaplan, M. (1999). *Spirituality, social support, and worry about health: Relationships in a sample of HIV+ women.* Manuscript submitted for publication.

Robbins, S. P., Canda, E. R., & Chatterjee, P. (1998). *Contemporary human behavior theory: A critical perspective for social work.* Boston: Allyn & Bacon.

Runnion, V. (undated). *Social Work Acuity Scale for Hospice.* Unpublished manuscript.

Russel, R. (1998). Spirituality and religion in graduate social work education. *Social Thought: Journal of Religion in the Social Services, 18*(2), 15-29.

Russel, R., Bowen, S., & Nickolaison, B. (2000). *Spiritually derived interventions in social work practice and education.* Paper presented at the Annual Program Meeting of the Council on Social Work Education, New York.

Sheridan, M., Bullis, R., Adcock, C., Berlin, S., & Miller, P. (1992). Practitioners' personal and professional attitudes and behaviors toward religion and spirituality: Issues for education and practice. *Journal of Social Work Education, 28*(2), 190-203.

Simon-Buller, S., Christopherson, V., & Jones, R. (1988-89). Correlates of sensing the presence of a deceased spouse. *Omega, 19*(1), 21-30.

Smith, D. (1993). Exploring the religious-spiritual needs of the dying. *Counseling and Values, 37,* 71-77.

Smith, E. (1995). Addressing the psychospiritual distress of death as reality: A transpersonal approach. *Social Work, 40*(3), 402-412.

Smith, E., & Gray, C. (1995). Integrating and transcending divorce: A transpersonal model. *Social Thought, 18*(1), 57-74.

Swett, L. (undated). *Spiritual shower.* Unpublished manuscript.

Wilber, K. (1980). *The Atman project: A transpersonal view of human development.* Wheaton, IL: Quest.

Wilber, K. (1993). (2nd ed.). *The spectrum of consciousness.* Wheaton, IL: Quest.

Wilber, K. (1995). *Sex, ecology, spirituality: The spirit of evolution.* Boston: Shambhala.

Wilber, K. (1996). *A brief history of everything.* Boston: Shambhala.

Worthington, E., & DiBlasio, F. (1990). Promoting mutual forgiveness within the fractured relationship. *Psychotherapy, 27,* 219-223.

York, G. (1987). Religious-based denial in the NICU: Implications for social work. *Social Work in Health Care, 12*(4), 31-45.

Transpersonal Social Work with Couples: A Compatibility-Intimacy Model

David Derezotes

SUMMARY. A model of transpersonal couple work is described, which builds upon Wilber's (1986) seminal theory of transpersonal development and Berne's (1961) Transactional Analysis Theory. A practical plan of assessment and intervention is forwarded. Essentially, the worker first assesses the primary level of consciousness of both partners and then develops a strategy to help both partners move more fluidly into their other two available (but currently underdeveloped) consciousness states. *[Article copies available for a fee from The Haworth Document Delivery Service: 1-800-342-9678. E-mail address: <getinfo@haworthpressinc.com> Website: <http://www.HaworthPress.com> © 2001 by The Haworth Press, Inc. All rights reserved.]*

KEYWORDS. Transpersonal, intimacy, couple, transactional analysis, social work

INTRODUCTION

In this article, a model of transpersonal couple work is described which builds upon Wilber's (1986) seminal theory of transpersonal development and

David Derezotes, PhD, LCSW, is Professor at the Graduate School of Social Work, University of Utah, Salt Lake City, UT 84112 (E-mail: Dderezotes@socwk. utah.edu).

[Haworth co-indexing entry note]: "Transpersonal Social Work with Couples: A Compatibility-Intimacy Model." Derezotes, David. Co-published simultaneously in *Social Thought* (The Haworth Press, Inc.) Vol. 20, No. 1/2, 2001, pp. 163-174; and: *Transpersonal Perspectives on Spirituality in Social Work* (ed: Edward R. Canda, and Elizabeth D. Smith) The Haworth Press, Inc., 2001, pp. 163-174. Single or multiple copies of this article are available for a fee from The Haworth Document Delivery Service [1-800-342-9678, 9:00 a.m. - 5:00 p.m. (EST). E-mail address: getinfo@haworthpressinc.com].

ego state theory from Transactional Analysis (Berne, 1961). Emphasis is placed upon the description of assessment and intervention strategies that the social work practitioner can incorporate into the personal helping style that she or he already uses.

First foreseen by Maslow (1971) as an emerging "Fourth Force" psychology of transcendence, transpersonalism is an inclusive theory that adds spirituality into mainstream psychology. Transpersonal practice thus seeks to assess and foster not only the spiritual, but also the cognitive, emotional, physical, and social dimensions of development (Cowley, 1993).

Transpersonalism is also a synthesizing theory that has room for many seemingly opposing viewpoints and perspectives. Transpersonalism offers a bridge between science and religion, two traditions that have been largely at odds with each other for centuries (Wilber, 1986). Transpersonal theory merges philosophies drawn from major psychological and religious traditions found across the world (Canda, 1991).

Although the literature provides some theory-based models of transpersonal practice, these models contain few practical guidelines for transpersonal assessment and intervention strategies with couples. For example, during the 1990s, a few best-selling books appeared that offered the public self-help approaches to fostering the spiritual aspects of love (e.g., Chopra, 1997; Moore, 1994). Textbooks have also been written that provide practitioners with theoretical frameworks of practice with couples or families that include the spiritual dimension (e.g., Brothers, 1992; Weinhold, 1989). Despite these advances, many counseling and social work students and practitioners have reported that they need more training in practical transpersonal assessment and intervention strategies (Derezotes, 1995; Derezotes & Evans, 1995).

Although there is growing evidence and consensus that transpersonalist theory has a legitimate place in social work practice with couples (Cowley, 1999), contributions in this critical area remain particularly sparse in social work curricula (Russel, 1998) and literature (Cowley & Derezotes, 1994). Transpersonal theory, although now over a quarter century old, has only recently been adopted by a few pioneers as a social work practice model (Cowley, 1993; Cowley, 1996). Recently, Cowley (1999) provided perhaps the most sophisticated description to date of how transpersonal theory might contribute to social work practice with couples.

A MODEL OF TRANSPERSONAL COUPLE WORK

Wilber's (1986) model of three phases of consciousness development provides the social worker with a framework that can help guide assessment and intervention with couples (as well as with individuals, families, and groups). The ego states used in Berne's (1961) Transactional Analysis (TA) Theory can be modified to build a simple model that the practitioner can use in assessing and intervening with couples.

From the TA perspective, when in relationship with each other, people can socially interact from any of three primary ego states. The *Child* (or C state) is that "part" of the person that acts like a child. Called the id by Freud (1913, 1921), the Child state is, therefore, primarily a self-oriented consciousness that is concerned about personal need, avoids pain, and pursues pleasure. The *Parent* (or P state) is that part that acts like a parent. Called the superego by Freud, the Parent state is a more other-oriented consciousness that is primarily concerned with the needs of others, that serves to protect others from pain and provide them with pleasure. In TA theory, the *Adult* serves like a referee, and watches and supervises the dialogue between the child and parent states. Called the ego by Freud, the Adult will be modified and relabeled the *Observing Self* (or OS state) in this article. It is thus the Observing self that is primarily concerned with transcending Child and Parent consciousness.

Three Levels of Consciousness

Wilber proposed that human consciousness can operate at three levels (see Figure 1). As illustrated, each phase has its own unique strengths that can contribute to a healthy relationship. Since any human strength held too rigidly can lead to difficulties, each level can also present potential challenges in a relationship.

Using the ego states described above, the *Prepersonal* phase can be understood as primarily Child consciousness. The Child dominates the Parent and Observing Self in the personality, so the C state is drawn larger than the P and OS in the figure. As illustrated, in Prepersonal consciousness, a person is able to play and experience pleasure and sensuality. However, that person could become so rigidly disconnected from and insensitive to others that he or she ignores his or her boundaries and becomes abusive or neglectful.

The *Personal* level can be understood as primarily Parent consciousness. The Parent dominates the Child and Observing Self, so the P state is drawn larger than the C and OS in the figure. As illustrated, in Personal consciousness, a person is able to be empathic and nurturing with others. However, the same people can become so rigidly disconnected from their own bodies (and thus "in their heads") that they ignore personal boundaries and allow themselves to be abused or neglected.

Finally, the *Transpersonal* level can be understood as primarily the consciousness of Observing Self. The Observing Self oversees the Child and Par-

FIGURE 1. Ego State Imbalances in Consciousness Levels

Level of Consciousness	Prepersonal	Personal	Transpersonal
Ego State Imbalance	(p) (os) (c)	(p) (os) (c)	(p) (os) (c)
Possible Relationship Strengths	Playful Sensuous	Empathic Nurturing	Peaceful Transcendent
Possible Relationship Inflexibilities	Body Focus Disconnected from Others	Mind Focus Disconnected from Body	Observer Focus Disconnected from World

Note: p = parent consciousness; os = observing self consciousness; c = child consciousness.

ent, so the OS state is drawn larger than the C and P in the figure. As illustrated, in transpersonal consciousness, a person may be able to develop a more peaceful and transcendent awareness. However, the same person could become so detached from the body and mind that one also becomes disconnected from the world one lives in.

Assessing Couples Using a Transpersonal Compatibility Model

Using the above description of the three phases of consciousness, a compatibility model of consciousness can be developed. Figure 2 shows three combinations of consciousness incompatibility in couple relationships. Each combination represents a relationship between two partners who live primarily in different levels of consciousness. As illustrated by the arrows in column two, each partner tends to relate from her or his dominant and comfortable consciousness level. The partners usually report being initially attracted to each other because their lovers have qualities (ego states) that remained underdeveloped in themselves.

Difficulty is experienced in the relationship when, instead of cultivating those underdeveloped ego states, each partner may become more rigidly attached to the dominant level of consciousness that they brought into the relationship. This imbalance often leads to deep unhappiness in both people because each is more willing to blame the other than to develop their own per-

FIGURE 2. Re-Balancing Ego States in Relationship

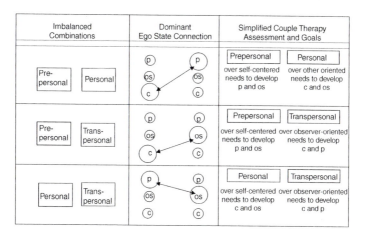

sonal wholeness. As this unhappiness continues, romance turns to power struggle and there is a tendency for both partners to refuse to change.

Column three in Figure 2 summarizes the work that clients may need to do, whether they stay in their relationship or not. The Prepersonal-dominant partner usually needs to further develop P and OS levels in order to move more fluidly between all the levels in her or his relationship and life. The Personal-dominant partner needs to further develop C and OS levels, and the Transpersonal-dominant partner needs to develop further C and P levels.

In the first combination, a Prepersonal-dominant person is coupled with a Personal-dominant person. The author sees this particular combination most frequently in his own practice (about 75% of cases). In this combination, both individuals may initially seem to agree that the needs of the Prepersonal-dominant partner are most important. However, if the Personal-dominant partner eventually develops better boundaries, the Prepersonal-dominant partner may react with abusiveness or other retaliation.

In the second most common combination, a Prepersonal-dominant person is coupled with a Transpersonal-dominant person. This combination may be found between two people with different social status roles, such as between a student and teacher or between a disciple and guru. The couple is suffering from what Wilber called the pre-trans fallacy in which the enthusiasm of prepersonal level functioning is mistaken for the transcendence of transpersonal functioning. As a result, each person can be seduced into giving his or her own power away to the partner. The Prepersonal-dominant person may not realize yet that his or her lover cannot also take the role of master or guru. The Transpersonal-dominant partner's gratification may be so intoxicating that he or she does not see how he or she is using the lover and neglecting his or her own spiritual path. As both become more unhappy, both tend to become more rigidly attached to their dominant levels of consciousness.

Finally, in the Personal-Transpersonal combination, the Personal-dominant person may be initially so attracted to the Transpersonal-dominant person's transcendence that he or she neglects his or her own spiritual path. Eventually, the Personal-dominant partner comes to resent that the lover does not reciprocate the caring he or she gives. The Transpersonal-dominant partner may enjoy being nurtured so much that she or he does not respond to the needs of the partner.

The model does not assume that differences in consciousness between partners are necessarily harmful to a relationship. In addition, compatibility is not so much about how similar people are as it is about how much people like and accept each other and can foster each other's multi-dimensional development. The combinations described in Figure 2 represent examples of how differences in ego states and consciousness levels can lead to developmental arrest. All areas of couple incompatibility are not described in this model. In addition, even when couples share similar levels of consciousness, there are still many interpersonal and intrapersonal challenges to deal with. Finally, the proportion of combinations seen in practice may change in the next decades: as our society ages and interest in spirituality increases, the number of individuals primarily functioning at the transpersonal level may enlarge.

Healing Is Wholing

A basic intervention goal is to help clients cultivate their underdeveloped ego states so that they can move between all three levels of consciousness with fluidity and purpose. As clients do this work, they are better able to either create more intimacy in the current relationship or to leave the relationship when there is insufficient compatibility for intimacy.

Thus, healing is wholing, i.e., to have all of one's parts. In this model, emphasis is placed upon each partner developing the ability to function at all three levels of consciousness. All three levels are equally important in facilitating individual and couple health. Each person needs to be able to function at the prepersonal level to enjoy a sensuous, sexual, playful life. Personal functioning is also important, since we all need to be able to care responsibly for ourselves and the people we love. Transpersonal functioning allows us to transcend identification with roles, possessions, status, wealth, and other attachments so that we can experience peace of mind and connection with our souls and the universe.

Clarifying Boundaries

Before couples can develop intimacy and move fluidly from one state of consciousness to another in their relationship, they need to learn about their own boundaries. In other words, each person learns how to talk with the partners about the limits of who they are and are not. In the beginning stage of intimacy, the romance in a relationship may easily obscure the differences between two partners. It is difficult for most people to quickly and accurately determine how compatible an attractive person might be to actually live with. As the partners learn how they are the same and how they are different, they can also assess how compatible they are and perhaps develop greater intimacy in their lives.

Multi-Dimensional Compatibility and Intimacy

Transpersonal theory *adds* spirituality to the dimensions of human compatibility and intimacy. Spirituality does *not replace* the other dimensions. Thus, partners assess their compatibility and build intimacy in the interrelated physical, emotional, cognitive, social, and spiritual dimensions of human development. Recognizing that each person has unique developmental landscapes, the social worker asks both partners to dialogue together about their compatibility in each of the five dimensions. Few couples are compatible in all dimensions, but both people may have basic needs that they consider essential to their happiness in a relationship.

Intimacy Building: Horizontal and Vertical

Intimacy is viewed in the model as having interrelated vertical and horizontal processes. *Vertical* intimacy has to do with building a body-mind-spirit connection within a person so that he or she is aware of all developmental dimensions. *Horizontal* intimacy occurs between two people who are sharing in the emotional, physical, cognitive, social, and spiritual dimensions. Many clients will seek the horizontal intimacy that seems to come when they first fall in love and will thus delay the hard work of developing their own vertical intimacy.

As both partners in a relationship develop vertical intimacy and experience the body-mind-spirit connection within themselves, their ability to connect with each other also broadens and deepens. Many clients want to change the pattern they find themselves in, but are unsure how to make such changes or even if such change is possible. The social worker can encourage clients to do the difficult internal work necessary to develop vertical intimacy.

Transferences and Countertransferences

Finally, in couple work interventions, effective processing of spiritual and religious transferences and countertransferences are particularly important. Practice in the spiritual dimension continuously challenges worker and client values and interpersonal reactions (Canda, 1989, 1988; Kilpatrick & Holland, 1990; Loewenberg, 1988; Siporin, 1985). Many clients draw from their religious beliefs when dealing with relationship issues. For example, most religions have doctrines or beliefs about extramarital sex and divorce.

The most effective social worker utilizes the tools of self-awareness and self-acceptance to deal with transference and countertransference. The social worker is aware of how the spiritual and religious beliefs held by clients and by oneself impact views of relationships. The worker is prepared to dialogue with clients about these beliefs so that clients can make informed choices about what kind of therapy they want.

For example, a married woman and man visit a social worker, asking for help with their very troubled relationship. The woman wants a divorce but her husband is a very religious man and believes that divorce is a sin and would destroy their lives. When the couple asks the social worker what she believes, the worker explains truthfully that she believes that divorce can sometimes be in the highest good. She tells the couple that she believes she can still work with them, but she understands if one or both of them wish to see another therapist who has different beliefs than she does.

CASE EXAMPLES

The interventions and case examples that follow illustrate a few of the methods that the author has used to help foster wholeness and healing with partners in relationships. These methods should be used only when there is sufficient safety in the relationship to do such work. Safety includes assurance that violence is under control in the relationship so that true dialogue can take place, because violence is usually a monologue that silences the victim. The methods that follow are adopted from psychodynamic, cognitive-behavioral, and experiential models (see Derezotes, 1995). The author has found that these interventions are most effective when combined (e.g., blending psychodynamic with experiential methods).

Psychodynamic

Psychodynamic methods ask clients to look at how their past experiences may still impact their present lives. The social worker can ask clients to do their own personal psychodynamic work openly in front of their partners. The goal is to help the clients better understand each other's past issues and related inner conflicts, which may now be obstacles to intimacy and love in the relationship. The social worker may also use the TA model to help clarify compatibility issues that surface.

For example, a social worker is seeing a gay couple with a Personal-dominant/Prepersonal-dominant combination who complain of frequent arguments and a loss of love. The worker may at some point in the sessions ask each man to draw a picture of his spiritual path, beginning with his family of origin and ending with their current relationship. The men then begin to get insight into how all their relationships are linked to their spiritual development. The social worker then diagrams for the couple their relationship, using TA ego states. The insights that the men gain seem to help them understand better why they are together and the work each needs to do. In this case, the Prepersonal-dominant man may focus on developing his parent ego state and the Personal-dominant man may focus on developing his child ego state.

Cognitive-Behavioral

In cognitive-behavioral interventions, the social worker can challenge clients to change their thinking or their behaviors related to the spiritual dimension. The worker may ask the clients to reframe the way they view the meaning of their relationship or their life. The worker may also ask the clients to replace old dysfunctional behaviors with new more functional behaviors that may foster their spirituality. Often, the worker asks the clients to define what behavioral changes they would like to see in themselves and their partners.

For example, a social worker is seeing a lesbian couple with a Transpersonal-dominant and Prepersonal-dominant combination; they complain of frequent arguments and a loss of love. The worker may at some point in the sessions ask each woman to view her partner as a spiritually wounded person who does not mean to harm them (rather than someone who is intentionally trying to hurt them). After this reframing, the worker might also then have the couple form a reciprocal contract in which each person agrees to change one behavior. The woman with a Transpersonal emphasis asks her partner to support her yoga training. In return, the woman with the Prepersonal emphasis agrees to take care of the bills each month.

Often such reciprocal contracting techniques are useful in evaluating progress with couples. Every week, each person can agree to change one specific behavior in return for a reciprocal change by the partner of one behavior. For example, John will come home earlier if Mary leaves him alone for an hour before they interact. If the couple is unable to agree upon a simple contract in the office, or if they are completely unable to have any mutual success at home with even a very simple contract, then the social worker considers the possibility of lack of commitment to the relationship or of more serious pathology in the relationship. A social worker might regularly try to leave couples with some kind of mutual agreement or other homework assignment at the end of each session. Typically, there are only 50 minutes of therapy time a week compared to usually over 100 hours of waking time between sessions that can be utilized by the clients.

Experiential

In experiential work, the social worker can strive to help clients become more aware and expressive of how they feel currently about themselves, their partners, and their relationships. There is much room for creativity. Often the worker has the clients express these feelings directly with each other. The expressions may be verbal or nonverbal (e.g., drawings, sculpture, psychodrama).

For example, a social worker is seeing a heterosexual couple who complains of frequent arguments and a loss of love. The worker may at some point in the sessions ask each partner to exaggerate the way they suspect their partner really wants them to act. The woman, who has a Personal level emphasis, gets down on her knees in mock drama and bows to her husband, saying, "Oh my patriarchal master, please forgive me for wanting to have a self. I am your obedient servant." They both laugh. Then the man, with a Prepersonal level emphasis, takes out his wallet and says, "Honey, here's a blank check for you, I am going to start working 100 hours a week so you can have all that you want. And anytime you want to process feelings, please let me know and I will listen..." The exercise "breaks the ice" for this couple and enables them to look at some deep spiritual issues in their marriage.

In another example, a worker might have a young couple talk about their last fight and examine what they felt (but had not yet directly expressed). The woman discovers that underneath her anger was fear of abandonment and a great deal of hurt about how her husband had ignored her since they were married. The man discovers that his anger is mostly about a fear of engulfment; he realizes that he has felt a loss of freedom and soul since his marriage.

The worker may also try to help the couple develop spiritual intimacy. Spiritual intimacy may be defined as the "sharing of souls" in which both partners experience a connectedness with the other's soul, with the world, and with each other. The social worker realizes that, no matter how well a couple communicates and handles conflicts, reads manuals on human sexuality, and follows the cognitive/behavioral tasks given to them by their social worker, without spiritual intimacy there may be an emptiness that cannot be filled. The worker strives to help clients become aware of their hunger for spiritual intimacy and of ways they might seek more of that kind of intimacy.

For example, a social worker is seeing a gay couple who complain of sexual dysfunction in their relationship. The couple has purchased self-help books, but all their knowledge and techniques do not seem to help. The worker asks the partners to try viewing their sexuality as a soul expression instead of a sexual dysfunction. After some dialogue and searching, the clients start to realize that they both feel alienated from each other. After they acknowledge the disconnection, they begin to develop a more soulful connection. Their sexuality also improves.

CONCLUSION

Work with couples is a very complex process, perhaps one of the most challenging areas of direct practice. The model presented in this article can be viewed as a beginning effort to apply Wilber's Transpersonal theory to this complex process. Future theorists will be challenged to consider such issues as (1) the interrelationship between couple work and individual spiritual work, (2) the role of the social worker in various phases of relationship such as pre-marital and post-divorce couple work, and (3) special considerations with diverse populations such as gay, lesbian, or transgendered people.

Because of this complexity, Transpersonal couple work may best be evaluated using both quantitative and qualitative methods. The best research may also be done by coalitions of social work practitioners and researchers in collaboration with their clients. Such collaborative efforts may not only help practitioners and clients make mid-course corrections in their own work, but also to ultimately add to the currently meager research literature in this practice area.

REFERENCES

Berne, E. (1961). *Transactional analysis in psychotherapy.* New York: Grove.
Brothers, B. J. (1992). *Spirituality and couples: Heart and soul in the therapeutic process.* New York: The Haworth Press, Inc.
Canda, E. R. (1988). Spirituality, religious diversity, and social work practice. *Social Casework, 69*(4), 238-247.
Canda, E. R. (1989). Religious content in social work education: A comparative approach. *Journal of Social Work Education, 25*(1), 36-45.
Canda, E. R. (1991). East/West Philosophical Synthesis in Transpersonal theory. *Journal of Sociology and Social Welfare (Dec.),* 21-23.

Chopra, D. (1997). *The path to love: Renewing the power of spirit in your life.* New York: Harmony Books.

Cowley, A. (1999). Transpersonal theory and social work practice with couples and families. *Journal of Family Social Work, 3*(2), 5-22.

Cowley, A. S. (1993). Transpersonal social work: A theory for the 1990s. *Social Work, 38*(5), 527-534.

Cowley, A. S. (1996). Transpersonal social work. In F. J. Turner (Ed.), *Social work treatment: Interlocking theoretical approaches* (pp. 663-698). New York: The Free Press.

Cowley, A. S., & Derezotes, D. S. (1994). Transpersonal psychology and social work education. *Journal of Social Work Education, 30*(1), 32-41.

Derezotes, D. S. (1995). Spiritual and religious factors in practice: Empirically-based recommendations for social work education. *Arete, 20*(1), 1-15.

Derezotes, D. S., & Evans, K. E. (1995). Spirituality and religiosity in practice: In-depth interviews of social work practitioners. *Social Thought: Journal of Religion in the Social Services, 18*(1), 39-56.

Freud, S. (1913). *Totem and taboo.* London: Hogarth Press.

Freud, S. (1921). *Massenpsychologie.* London: Hogarth Press.

Kilpatrick, A. C., & Holland, T .P. (1990). Spiritual dimensions of practice. *The Clinical Supervisor, 8*(2), 125-140.

Loewenberg, F. M. (1988). *Religion and social work practice in contemporary American society.* New York: Columbia University Press.

Maslow, A. H. (1971). *The further reaches of human nature.* New York: The Viking Press.

Moore, T. (1994). *Soul Mates: Honoring the mysteries of love and relationship.* New York: Harper Collins.

Russel, R. (1998). Spirituality and religion in graduate social work education. In E. R. Canda (Ed.), *Spirituality in social work: New directions* (pp. 15-29). Binghamton, NY: Haworth Pastoral Press.

Siporin, M. (1985). Current social work perspectives on clinical practice. *Clinical Social Work Journal, 13*(3), 198-217.

Weinhold, B. (1989). Transpersonal theories in family treatment. In D. Fennel & B. Weinhold (Eds.), *Counseling families.* Denver: Love Publishing Company.

Wilber, K. (1986). The spectrum of development, the spectrum of psychopathology, and treatment modalities. In K. Wilber, J. Engler, & D. Brown (Eds.), *Transformations of consciousness: Conventional and contemplative perspectives on development* (pp. 65-159). Boston: New Science Library.

Index